S

DICTIONARY
OF
SPEECH & HEARING

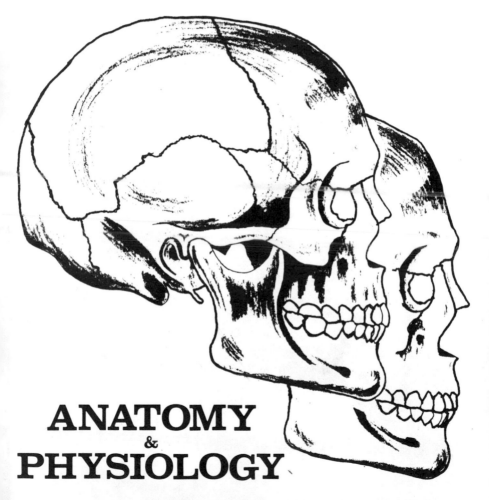

ANATOMY
&
PHYSIOLOGY

Joseph F. Brown

Library of Congress Catalog Card Number: 74-76789

ISBN   0-914592-02-5 Cloth Edition
ISBN   0-914592-01-7 Paper Edition

Cover Design and Illustrations
by
Alys Fuel

Speech and Hearing Service
P. O. Box 26361
Sacramento, Ca 95826

PRINTED IN THE UNITED STATES OF AMERICA

Preface
to the first edition

This book has been written with the object of providing a survey of human speech and hearing anatomy and physiology terms compiled for the first time in this form. In a single volume are terms which have heretofore appeared only in scattered books, periodicals and journals.

Every book is the product of an idea, and for this I am indebted to Marjorie Sellers, librarian, Park College, Kansas City, Missouri. I wish to express appreciation to all those who have aided in the preparation of this book , in particular Kathie Hefner for her valuable comments and suggestions.

Joseph F. Brown

A

Å: (ANGSTROM UNIT) Anders J. Angstrom, Swedish Physicist. Unit of wavelength of corpuscular or electromagnetic radiations. Equal to one hundred-millionth of a centimeter; 10^{-8}cm.

ABARTHROSIS: A free moving joint or a point where bones move freely on each other.

ABDOMINAL APONEUROSIS: A broad flat sheet of tendinous tissue in the anterior abdominal wall from the pubic bone to the sternum bone. The midline portion is a dense fibrous band, the linea alba which extends from the pubic symphysis up to the ensiform process of the sternum bone. It divides on each side of the linea alba into two layers, one deep and one superficial to the rectus abdominis muscle. The superficial layer attaches superiorly to the lower portion of the pectoralis major muscle, ensiform process of the sternum bone and joining costal cartilage. It attaches inferiorly to the anterior iliac spine and pubic symphysis.

ABDOMEN: The portion of the body between the thorax and pelvis.

ABDOMINAL MUSCLES: Consist of the external oblique, internal oblique, rectus abdominis and transverse abdominis.

ABDUCENTS: To draw away from the midline.

ABDUCENTS NERVE: (ABDUCENT NERVE) VI cranial, a motor nerve with its origin at the inferior border of the basal surface of the pons, entering the orbit through the superior orbital fissure and terminating in the lateral muscle of the eye.

ABDUCENS NUCLEUS: A group of nerve cells in the fourth ventricle of the brain from which the abducent (VI cranial) nerve rises.

ABDUCT: To draw away from the midline.

ABDUCTOR MUSCLE: A muscle which draws away from the midline.

ABSCESS: An area of pus contained within a cavity, surrounded by inflamed tissue.

ABSCISSA: The horizontal line or X axis on a graph showing the relationship of two values, such as date and time.

ACCESSORY NERVE: (ACCESSORIUS NERVE) XI cranial, a motor nerve with the cranial portion originating from the nucleus ambigious which exits from the medulla oblongata by rootlets. It is directed laterally through the jugular foramen and directed to the levator veli palatini muscle and uvula and then directed to the vagus (X cranial) nerve following the course of the recurrent nerve. The spinal portion has its origin in the spinal cord anterior horn and exit as nerves (cranial one through four or five) joining to form a single nerve directed along the spinal cord throu through the occipital bone foramen magnum into the cranium following the cranial portion and exiting through the jugular foramen. At this point it joins fibers of the cranial portion and directed to the sternocleidomastoid and trapezius muscles.

ACCESSORY SINUSES: (PARANASAL SINUSES) The ethmoidal, frontal, maxillary and sphenoidal sinuses of the nose lined with ciliated mucous membrane.

ACETABULUM: Rounded cavity on the external surface of the os coxae (hip bone) into which the femur bone head fits.

ACETYLCHOLINE: A acid ester of choline at muscle endplates and parasympathetic fibers which functions in transmission of an impulse across a synaptic gap or junction from one nerve fiber to another. It is quickly destroyed by acetylcholinerase; abbreviation-ACh.

ACh: Abbreviation for acetylcholine.

ACICULAR: Shaped like a needle; needle pointed.

ACINIFORM: Shaped like a grape.

ACOUSTIC: Pertaining to hearing or sound.

ACOUSTIC CELL: A hair cell in the organ of Corti in the inner ear.

ACOUSTIC CENTER: (ACOUSTIC CORTEX) Area in the temporal lobe of the cerebrum which serves as the terminal center for the nerve fibers in the inner ear conducting nerve impulses toward the center.

ACOUSTIC CREST: (AMPULLARIS CRISTA) A thick portion in the lining of the ampulla through which fibers of the vestibular nerve, a division of the auditory (VIII cranial) nerve, pass to the hair cells.

ACOUSTIC IMPEDANCE: (ACOUSTIC REFLEX) A protective mechanism of the tympanic cavity (middle ear) intervated by the facial (VII cranial) nerve in response to either sound at approximately 70-90 dB sensation level depending on the frequency or tactile stimulus. The reflex is caused by the stapeduis muscle pulling the stapes(stirrup) bone footplate laterally and the tensor tympanic muscle pulling the malleus (hammer) bone attached to the tympanic membrane (eardrum) inward. These contractions increase the stiffness of the ossicular chain with a result of mechanical dampening of tone sensitivity as much as 20 dB.

ACOUSTIC TUBERCLE: (TUBERCULUM) The dorsal nucleus of the cochlea nerve.

ACQUIRED: Obtained after birth; not inherited. 2. Learned through experience.

ACROMEGALY: Chronic enlargement of bone and soft tissue of the face, feet or hands, due to excessive secretion of the pituitary gland.

ACROMICLAVICULAR: The acromion and clavicle bone.

ACROMION: The triangular lateral projection of the scapula forming the shoulder joint which articulates with the clavicle bone.

ACTION POTENTIAL: (AFTER POTENTIAL) Changes in electrical potential that occurs at the surface of muscle or nervous tissue at the moment of excitation.

ACUSTICUS: The acoustic (vestibulocochlearis) VIII cranial nerve.

ACUSTICUS INTERNUS MEATUS: A canal in the temporal bone petrous portion for passage of the acoustic (VIII cranial) and facial (VII cranial) nerves.

ACUTE: Of sudden onset and short duration; as in acute pain.

ADAM'S APPLE: (THYROID CARTILAGE) The shield shaped cartilage in the larynx formed by the two thyroid cartilage laminae.

ADAPTATION: The ability of a part or structure to adjust to a change in its environment.

ADDUCTION: Movement toward the midline.

ADDUCTOR MUSCLE: A muscle which draws toward the midline.

ADENOIDS: (PHARYNGEAL TONSIL) A mass of lymphoid tissue on the posterior wall of the nasopharynx.

ADIPOSE: Pertaining to fat. 2. To be fat.

ADIPOSE TISSUE: A form of areolar tissue with densely packed cells containing fat. The cells are large and sphere-shaped.

ADITUS: The designation of an entrance.

ADITUS AD ANTRUM: Recess leading from the attic of the tympanic cavity (middle ear) to the mastoid cavity. The malleus (hammer) bone head and the majority of the incus (anvil) bone are in the attic area.

ADITUS AD INFUNDIBULUM: A canal from the third ventricle of the brain into the infundibulm.

ADITUS GLOTTIDIS INFERIOR: The inferior entrance into the glottis.

ADITUS GLOTTIDIS SUPERIOR: The superior entrance into the glottis.

ADITUS LARYNGIS: The triangular superior opening into the vestibule of the larynx by which it communicates with the pharynx. The entrance is wide in front, narrow behind and sloping obliquely backward and downward.

ADORAL: Near or toward the mouth.

ADRENALIN: A hormone (epinephrine) secreted by the ectodermal medulla of the adrenal glands.

ADRENAL GLANDS: Ductless glands of the endocrine system located at the superior pole of each kidney. The right is triangular shaped, the left semilunar shaped. Each gland is covered by a thin capsule, the cortex and the central portion is the medulla. The cortex consist of a network of connective tissue. The medulla secreates epinephrine.

ADRENALINE: (EPINEPHRINE) A hormone produced by the adrenal gland medulla portion. The effect is like those produced by the sympathetic division of the autonomic nervous system.

AFFERENT FIBER: Carrier of incoming impulses to nerve cells.

AFFERENT NEURON: A sensory neuron conducting a impulse from a receptor toward the brain or spinal cord.

AFTER HEARING: Auditory sensation still present after the stimulus creating the sensation has ceased.

AFTER POTENTIAL: (ACTION POTENTIAL) Changes in electrical potential that occurs at the surface of muscle or nervous tissue at the moment of excitation.

AIR: Consist of a mixture of gases that are odorless, invisible and tasteless. Air contains 0.8 percent argon, 78 percent nitrogen, 21 percent oxygen, aqueous vapor, carbon dioxide and traces of ammonia, helium, krypton, neon xenon and other rare gases.

AIR CELL: A cavity in bones of the cranium which contains air; such as the ethmoid bone sinus.

AIR EXCHANGE: Exchange of air at a rate of approximately twenty times a minute at rest. When movement increases, rate increases to approximately twenty to thirty times per minute.

AIR SAC: (ALVEOLAR SAC) The termination point of an air passage within the lung. The lung wall is pitted with pocketlike structures (alveolus) and each sac is connected to a respiratory bronchiole by an alveolar duct. Each air cell contains a network of capillaries where red blood cells make the carbon dioxide for oxygen exchange.

AIRWAY: The natural passage for air in the body.

ALA: A structure that is winglike. pl. alae,

ALA AURIS: The pinna or the external portion of the ear.

ALA OF ETHMOID BONE: Small projection on each side of the ethmoid bone.

ALA OF ILIUM: The wide upper portion of the os ilium or the iliac bone.

ALA MAJOR OSSIS SPHENOIDALIS: (GREAT WING OF SPHENOID) The large wing shaped process process on each side of the sphenoid bone body. The cerebral portion forms the anterior of the floor of the middle cranial fossa; the orbital portion forming the lateral wall of the orbit.

ALA MINOR OSSIS SPHENOIDALIS: (SMALL WING OF SPHENOID)
A triangular plate of bone extending both laterally and horizontally from the anterior of the body. It forms a portion of the cranial fossa and roof of the orbit and articulates with the frontal bone.

ALA NASI: The lower extended flared portion of the outer side of each nostril.

ALA VOMERIS: One of the two lateral extensions of bone on the vomer bone anterior border.

ALAR: Pertaining to a wing or ala.

ALAR LAMINA: (ALAR PLATE) In embryo development, either of the longitudinal zones of the neural tube from which the dorsal gray columns of the spinal cord and sensory portions of the brain develope.

ALIZARIN: A red dye obtained from coal tar.

ALLANTOIS: In embryo development, a tubular elongated bladder between the amnion and chorion.

ALL-OR-NONE PRINCIPLE: Proposes that a stimulus either strong or weak initiates a nerve impulse will be the same as an impulse initiated from a stronger stimulus. A nerve impulse travels its course with constant energy.

ALPHA NERVE FIBERS: (GROUP A FIBERS) The largest of the anterior horn motor cells of the somatic nervous system with a conduction speed of approximately one hundred meters per second.

ALVEOLAR ARCH: The arch formed by the alveolar process of either jaw.

ALVEOLAR BONE: The bone of the alveolar process of the mandible and maxillae bones.

ALVEOLAR BORDER: The upper surface of the mandible hollowed into cavities for the teeth.

ALVEOLAR CANAL: (DENTAL CANAL) The canals in the maxilla bone for the communication of blood vessels and nerves to the upper teeth.

ALVEOLAR CAVITY: A tooth socket in either of the jaw bones.

ALVEOLAR DUCT: A branch of a bronchiole which leads to the alveolar sacs of the lungs.

ALVEOLAR PROCESS-MANDIBLE BONE: The superior border of the mandible bone, containing cavities for the lower teeth.

ALVEOLAR PROCESS-MAXILLA BONE: The inferior border of the maxilla bone containing cavities for the upper teeth.

ALVEOLAR SAC: (AIR SAC) The termination point of an air passage within the ling. The lung wall is pitted with pocketlike structures (alveolus) and each sac is connected to a respiratory bronchiole by an alveolar duct. Each air cell contains a network of capillaries where red blood cells make the carbon dioxide for oxygen exchange.

ALVEOLARIS LIMBUS: (ARCUS ALVEOLARIS) The superior edge of the mandible bone alveolar process. 2. The superior edge of the maxilla bone alveolar process.

ALEOLI PUMONIS: The small depressions in the alveolar sacs through the wall of which the carbon dioxide (CO_2) and oxygen (O) exchange is made.

ALVEOLUS: An air cell in the lung. 2. A little hollow. 3. A tooth socket. pl. alveoli.

AMELOBLAST: (ENAMEL BUILDER) Cylinder shaped epithelial cell in the tooth enamel, the innermost layer from which enamel is made.

AMNION: (AMNIONIC MEMBRANE) In embryo development, the membrane surrounding the embryo containing the thin watery amniontic fluid in which the embryo is covered.

AMNIOTIC CAVITY: Developed in the embryo stage by cells around the cavity within the ectoderm. The cells form a thin vesicle, the amnion; with a cavity formed, the amniotic cavity.

AMORPHOUS: Without a distinct form. 2. Shapless.

AMPHIARTHROSIS: Slightly movable joints throughout the body, permitting some movement. There are two types; symphysis, where the bone surfaces are connected by a broad flat disk of fibrocartilaqe and synohondrosis, a temporary joint where the cartilage is changed to bone before adult life.

AMPLITUDE: A measurement of vibratory motion; the maximum displacement of a body from equilibrium equal to half the total of vibratory motion.

AMPULLA: An enlarged portion of the semicircular canal where it connects with the vestibule of the inner ear. It contains sense organs (hair cells) that when excited by movement of the waterlike fluids in the canals transmit nerve impulses to the brain. pl. ampullae.

AMPULLAE OF SEMICIRCULAR DUCTS: The small expanded area of the semicircular ducts near the junction with the utricle where the crista ampullaris is present.

AMPULLARIS CRISTA: (ACOUSTIC CREST) A thick portion in the lining of the ampulla through which fibers of the vestibular nerve, a division of the auditory (VIII cranial) nerve, pass to the hair cells.

AMYGDALOID: Almond-shaped; tonsil like.

AMYGDALOID BODY: (AMYGDALOID NUCLEUS) A almond shaped mass of gray matter in the roof of the lateral ventricle.

AMYGDALOID FOSSA: The depression for the tonsil between the pillars of fauces.

ANAPHASE: The third phase in mitosis (cell division) between metaphase and telephase when the group of daughter chromosomes separate and migrate toward the poles.

ANASTOMOSE: To open or join one into another;such as arteries to veins.

ANATOMICAL PLANES: The three planes of the body; coronal (frontal), sagittal and transverse.

PLANE	DIRECTION OF PLANE	DIVIDING INTO
Coronal (frontal)	Side-to-Side(lateral)	Front and Back parts
Sagittal	Front-to-Back	Right and Left parts
Transverse(horizontal)	Horizontal(across)	Upper and lower parts

ANATOMICAL POSITION: The body standing erect, arms at the side, eyes, head and palms of hands are forward.

ANDERNACH'S OSSICLES: Johnn W. von Andernach, German Physician. The tiny bones found in the cranial sutures.

ANDROGEN: Male sex hormone which produces functional and structural changes at puberty.

ANEROID: Containing no liquid. 2. Dry.

ANEROID BAROMETER: A barometer that, due to the movement of atmospheric pressure in bending a metalic surface, is made to move a pointer.

ANGIOLOGY: The study of blood and lymph vessels.

ANGLE: The area or space near the line or point where two lines or planes meet.

ANGLE-MANDIBLE BONE: The point where the posterior border of the mandible bone ramus meets the inferior border of the mandible bone body.

ANGLE'S CLASSIFICATION SYSTEM: Edward H. Angle, American Orthodontist. A system for classification of facial bone malocclusions based on lower and upper jaw relationship, divided into the following classes: Class I- Normal jaw relationship with abdnormal teeth position(neutroclusion). Class II- A retruded mandible bone in relation to the maxilla bone (distoclusion). Class III- A protuded mandible bone in relation to the maxilla bone (mesioclusion). Class IV-One half of the dental arch being in distal occlusion on the lateral half of the mouth and in mesial occlusion on the other half.

ANGSTROM UNIT; Symbol A. Anders J. Angstrom, Swedish Physicist. Unit of wavelength of corpuscular or electromagnetic radiations. Equal to one hundred-millionth of a centimeter; 10^{-8}cm.

ANGIIIAR: Bent sharply. 2. Having angles or corners.

ANGULAR GYRUS: On the inferior parietal lobe of the brain over the posterior end of the superior temporal sulcus.

ANGULAR VELOCITY: Term applied to rotational motion; the vector whose magnitude is the time rate of change of the angle Θ rotated through w=Θ dt.

ANIMAL POLE: In embryo development the location across from the yolk where polar bodies are formed and pinched off.

ANION: An ion carrying a negative (-) charge. It is attracted by, and travels to, the positive (+) pole.

ANLAGE: (PRIMORDIUM) In embryo development, the earliest accumulation of cells which constitute the beginning of a future part, organ or tissue.

ANNULAR: In the shape of a ring.

ANNULAR CARTILAGE: A ring-shaped cartilage which holds the tympanic membrane (eardrum) in place.

ANNULAR LIGAMENT: A fibrous ring which holds the stapes (stirrup) bone footplate in the fenestra vestibuli (oval window) of the tympanic cavity (middle ear).

ANNULUS: A ring shaped structure. 2. ring. pl. annuli.

ANNULUS TYMPANICUS: (TYMPANIC RING) A fibrocartilaginous ring forming a portion of the temporal bone which develops into the pare tympanica of the bone by which the tympanic membrane (eardrum) is held in place.

ANODE: The positive (+) pole of an electrical source.

ANOMALY: Deviation from the normal.

ANOXIA: Deprivation of oxygen in the blood.

ANSA: A structure in the form of a arc or loop. pl. ansae.

ANSA CERVICALIS: (ANSA HYPOGLOSSI) A loop of nerves which exit the hypoglossal (XII cranial) nerve, at the level of the cricoid cartilage and directed to the omo hyoid, sternohyoid and sternothyroid muscles.

ANSIFORM: Shaped like a loop.

ANTAGONIST: Muscle which contracts with and limits the action of an agonist with which it is paired. 2. A tooth in one jaw that fits with a tooth in the opposite jaw.

ANTAGONISTIC: The ability of a muscle to oppose or resist the action, or the effect, of another muscle.

ANTERIOR: Term for direction, toward the front.

ANTERIOR AURICULAR NERVE BRANCHES: Sensory branches of the auriculotemporal nerve, a branch of the mandibular nerve, the third and largest division of the trigeminal (V cranial) nerve directed to the external ear helix and tragus.

ANTERIOR CENTRAL GYRUS: A gyrus on the border of the central sulcus containing motor nerve cells.

ANTERIOR CEREBRAL COMMISSURE: A band of fibers which pass through the lamina terminalis connecting the cerebral hemispheres.

ANTERIOR COLUMN: (ANTERIOR HORN)(VENTRAL HORN) The gray matter of the spinal cord, wider than the dorsal horn, containing cells associated with motor functioning.

ANTERIOR LIGAMENT OF THE MALLEUS BONE: (MALLEI ANTERIOR LIGAMENT) A band of fiber, one end attached to the malleus (hammer) bone neck, with the other end attached to the tympanic cavity (middle ear) anterior wall.

ANTERIOR MEDIAL FISSURE: (VENTRAL MEDIAL FISSURE) The deeper of the two divisions which divide the spinal cord into left and right halves. It contains a double fold of pia mater with the floor formed by the ventral white commissure.

ANTERIOR NASAL SPINE: A sharp process on the nasal crest portion of the maxilla bone.

ANTERIOR PILLAR OF FAUCES: (GLOSSOPALATINE ARCH)(PALATO-GLOSSAL ARCH) The anterior of the two folds of mucous membrane formed by the downward curve from the soft palate to the side of the tongue base, enclosing the palatoglossal muscle.

ANTERIOR PROCESS-MALLEUS BONE: A delicate spine-like process at the junction of the neck and manubrium process.

ANTERIOR SUPERIOR ALVEOLAR NERVE BRANCH: A sensory branch of the maxillary nerve, the second division of the trigeminal (V cranial) nerve directed to the maxillary sinus and nasal cavity floor.

ANTERIOR SURFACE-MAXILLA BONE: The area forward and lateral containing the landmarks of the anterior nasal spine, canine eminence and fossa, incisive fossa and infraorbital foramen.

ANTERiOR TRANSVERSE TEMPORAL GYRUS: The auditory area of the temporal lobe, area 4l.

ANTERIOR WALL: (CAROTID WALL) The anterior wall of the tympanic cavity (middle ear). It is wider at the top than the bottom, with a thin plate of bone seperating it from the carotid canal. The top portion of the wall is perforated by the tendon for support of the tensor tympani muscle and the opening of the auditory tube (Eustachian). They are seperated by a thin horizonal plate of bone; the sepum canalis musculotubarii.

ANTHROPOID: To resemble man.

ANTIDURETIC HORMONE: (ADH) Controls water and electrolyte balance of body fluids. Secretion is from cells in the hypothalamus.

ANTIHELIX: The inner semicircular ridge of the cartilage, above the concha and in front of the helix, or outer cartilage of the external ear.

ANTILOBIUM: The tagus, a small stiff ridge in front of the external ear opening.

ANTITRAGICUS MUSCLE: An intrinsic muscle of the external ear. ORIGIN-Outer portion of the antitragus. INSERTION-The antihelix. NERVE- Facial (VII cranial), posterior auricular branch.

ANTITRAGUS: A small projection on the cartilagous ridge opposite the tragus, below the antihelix of the external ear.

ANTROTYMPANIC: The mastoid antrum and tympanic cavity (middle ear).

ANTRUM: Cavity or hollow space, usually cavities located in bones. pl. antrums, antra.

ANTRUM AURIS: The external auditory canal.

ANTRUM OF HIGHMORE: (MAXILLARY SINUS) A large pyramid shaped cavity in the maxilla bone body. The apex extends into the zygomatic process and the base is formed by the nasal cavity lateral wall. It communicates with the middle passage of the nasal cavity on the same side. They appear from the fourth month of fetal life and are developed fully by puberty.

ANVIL: (INCUS BONE) The middle of the three bones of the tympanic cavity (middle ear) which articulates with the malleus (hammer) bone by a diarthrodial joint. It consist of the body and two pro-cesses.

AORTIC HIATUS: Opening in the diaphragm, at the level of the twelfth thoracic vertebra, through which the aorta passes from the abdomen to the thorax.

APERIODIC: An occurence which is not consistent.

APEX: The top of a organ or structure. 2. The top of the arytenoid cartilage directed backward and medial.

APICIS DENTIS FOREMAN: Opening near the top of the tooth root for passage of blood vessels and nerves which supply the pulp.

APICAL FORAMEN: The opening at the tooth root for passage of blood vessels and nerves.

APONEUROSIS: A sheet of fibrous connective tissue which attaches bone to muscle, or muscle to muscle. pl. aponeuroses.

APPENDICULAR SKELETON: Bones of the limbs; such as the pectoral (upper) and pelvic (lower) girdles.

APPENDIX: The extention of a structure that acts as an appendage. pl. appendixes.

APPENDIX OF THE LARYNGEAL VENTRICLE: (LARYNGEAL SACCULE) (VENTRICULAR APPENDIX) A membranous sac located between the inner surface of the thyroid cartilage and thyroarytenoid muscle. This saccule is enclosed by a capsule of fibrous tissue. The ary-epiglottis muscle (Hilton muscle) is next to the saccule. The origin at the arytenoid cartilage apex becomes less defined and inserts on the lateral margin of the epiglottis. The muscle compresses the sac and from the viscous glands on its surface a secretion lubri-cates the true vocal fold surfaces.

APPOSITION: The fitting of adjacent parts.

APPROXIMATION: An action that brings two or more structures in-to an adjoining position, but not exactly correct.

Aq: Abbreviation for water.

AQUEDUCT: A canal or passage in an organ or structure.

AQUEDUCT OF FALLOPII: (FACIAL CANAL) A canal through which the facial (VII cranial) nerve passes, located in the temporal bone petrous portion. It is directed between the cochlea and semicircular canals, coursing above the fenestra vestibuli (oval window) then down along the area of mastoid air cells to the stylomastoid foramen, continuing to divide into two branches at the posterior border of the mandible bone ramus.

AQUEDUCT OF SYLVIUS: (CEREBRAL AQUEDUCT) Jacobus Sylvius, French Anatomist. A narrow canal from the third to the fourth ventricle of the brain through which cerebrospinal fluid passes.

ARACHNOID: Being web-like.

ARACHNOID CAVITY: The space between the arachnoid membrane and dura mater; or, the space between the arachnoid membrane and the pia mater.

ARACHNOID LAYER: (ARACHNOID MATER) (ARACHNOID MEMBRANE) The middle of the three layers covering the brain and spinal cord. A vascular delicate layer between the dura mater and pia mater.

ARCH OF CRICOID: The narrow anterior portion of the cricoid cartilage.

ARCIFORM: Curved or arch shaped.

ARCUATE: Shaped like a arch; or bow shaped.

ARCUATE CREST: A ridge directed horizontally which seperates the depressions on the arytenoid cartilage.

ARCUATE EMINENCE: An arch shaped prominence on the temporal bone petrous portion under which the superior semicircular canal is located.

ARCUS ALVEOLARIS: (ALVEOLARIS LIMBUS) The superior edge of the mandible bone alveolar process. 2. The superior edge of the maxilla bone alveolar process.

AREA: A specific portion of an organ or structure.

AREA 4: (MOTOR AREA) The area of motor impulses anterior to the frontal lobe central sulcus forming a band from the lateral fissure to the dorsal border of the hemisphere. The left portion of the band controls body right side action with the larynx and tongue controlled by the lower portion of the band.

AREA 41: (TRANSVERSE TEMPORAL GYRUS) (HESCHL'S GYRUS) Richard L. Heschl, Austrian Physician. The auditory reception center below the Sylvius fissure of the temporal lobe.

AREA 44-45: (BROCA'S AREA) (SPEECH CENTER) Pierre P. Broca, French Surgeon. The area on the left side of the brain in the inferior frontal gyrus rostal to the motor area (area 8) for motor speech.

AREOLA: A very small space in tissue. 2. Mesh-like organization of tissue in various spaces in the body. pl. areolae.

AREOLAR TISSUE: (LOOSE CONNECTIVE TISSUE) Consist of cells in an irregular net like structure of fibers. It forms the "bed" for mucous membrane and skin, and surrounds blood vessels and nerves.

AXILLA: (ARMPIT) The small hollow under the arm. pl. axillae.

ARTHRODIA JOINT: (GLIDING JOINT) A type of diarthrodial joint where the articular surfaces are alternately concave and convex.

ARTHROLOGY: The study of joints.

ARTICULAR: of, or relating to a joint.

ARTICULAR CAPSULE: A fibrous band enclosing the articulation of the inferior cornu (horn) of the thyroid, with the cricoid cartilage on each side.

ARTICULAR CARTILAGE: Hyaline cartilage covering the articular surfaces of bones.

ARTICULAR CONDYLE: Either of the round projections on each side of the occipital bone foramen magnum for articulation with the atlas; the first cervical vertebra.

ARTICULAR DISK: An oval thin plate between the condyle of the mandible bone and the mandibular fossa dividing the joint into two cavities.

ARTICULAR EMINENCE OF THE TEMPORAL BONE: A round shaped eminence which forms the glenoid fossa anterior boundary.

ARTICULAR FACET: A smooth surface on a bone for articulation with another structure.

ARTICULAR NERVE BRANCHES: Sensory branches of the auriculo-temporal nerve, a branch of the mandibular nerve, the third and largest division of the trigeminal (V cranial) nerve directed to the temporomandibular joint.

ARTICULAR TUBERCLE: A round cartilage covered elecation of the temporal bone zygomatic process. It forms the anterior border of the mandibular fossa.

ARTICULATE: A joint or juncture of bones. 2. Movement and place-ment of the articulators during speech production. 3. To express clearly or effectively.

ARTICULATOR MOVEMENT: Movement of the various structures of the mouth.

ARTICULATORS: The hard and soft palate, lips, teeth and tongue responsible for modification of acoustic properties of the vocal tract.

ARYEPIGLOTTIC FOLDS: Folds of mucous membrane which enclose ligaments and muscle fibers stretched between the arytenoid carti-lage apex and the side of the epiglottis forming the entrance to the larynx.

ARYEPIGLOTTICIS MUSCLE: (HILTON MUSCLE) John Hilton, English Surgeon. Muscle fibers located next to the laryngeal saccule. Its origin is the arytenoid apex, becoming less defined and inserting on the epiglottis lateral surface. Its action compresses the saccule whose secretion lubricates the surface of the true vocal folds.

ARYTENOID ANGLES: Anterior angle; located near the arytenoid base as a near pointed projection, the vocal process, for the insertion of the vocal ligament. The posterior-lateral angle; near the base pro-jects and is thick, forming the muscular process for attachment for the lateral and posterior cricoarytenoid muscles.

ARYTENOID APEX: The top of each arytenoid cartilage topped by a small cartilaginous conical nodule, the corniculate cartilage.

ARYTENOID CARTILAGE: The pair of hyaline cartilages located on the superior border of the cricoid lamina at the back of the larynx. Each is pyramidal in form and consists of an apex and four surfaces.

ARYTENOID MUSCLE: An intrinsic adductor on the posterior surface of the arytenoid cartilages. ORIGIN AND INSERTION- Posterior surface and lateral border of one arytenoid cartilage, and inserting into the same area of the opposite arytenoid cartilage. A complex muscle designated as two portions, the oblique and transverse arytenoid muscles.

ARYTENOID OBLIQUE MUSCLE: The most superficial of the two parts of the arytenoid muscle. ORIGIN- Arytenoid cartilage muscular process. INSERTION- Apex of opposite arytenoid cartilage. ACTION- Close the inlet of the larynx. NERVE-Vagus (X cranial), laryngeal and recurrent branches.

ARYTENOID TRANSVERSE MUSCLE: The deepest part of the arytenoid muscle. ORIGIN- Arytenoid cartilage muscular process. DIREC- TION- Horizontal. INSERTION- Lateral margin and posterior surface of the apex of the opposite cartilage. ACTION- Brings the arytenoid cartilages together. NERVE- Vagus (X cranial), laryngeal and recurrent branches.

ARYVOCALIS MUSCLE: A bundle of small fibers inserting into the vocal ligament.

ASSOCIATION FIBERS: Fibers of two types; long fibers formed into specific bundles interconnecting areas of the hemisphere, and short fibers which connect gyri of the hemisphere located under the gray matter of the cortex.

ASSOCIATION NEURON: (INTERNUNCIAL NEURON) A central neuron being both afferent and efferent in mediating impulses between a motor and sensory neuron.

ASTHENIA: Being slender with slight muscular development. 2. Weakness, or lack of energy.

ASTHENIC: (BREATHY) Vocal quality due to the incomplete blockage of the air passage. It is most noticeable at the beginning of the expiratory cycle and limits the range of intensity due to organically caused, or poor vocal habits.

ASTROCYTE: (SPIDER CELL) A neuroglia cell, star shaped with many branching processes.

ATAVISM: Reversion or occurence of a characteristic not found in more immediate ancestor, or in direct line.

ATLAS: The first cervical vertebra, located in the neck.

ATMOSPHERIC PRESSURE: Air pressure exerted by the atmosphere.

ATRIUM: A chamber or space in the ear, lung or larynx. pl. atria.

ATTENUATE: Tapering to a long thin point.

ATTIC: (EPITYMPANIC RECESS) (RECESSUS EPITYMPANICUS) The superior portion of the tympanic cavity (middle ear) above the tympanic membrane (eardrum) containing the malleus (hammer) bone head and the incus (anvil) bone short limb.

ATTRITION: To wear down by friction. 2. Rubbing together.

AUDITORY ACUITY: Sensitivity to sound.

AUDITORY AREA: The transverse temporal gyrus (area 41) below the Sylvius fissure of the temporal lobe, the auditory reception center.

AUDITORY CANAL-EXTERNAL: The passage leading from the external ear to the tympanic membrane (eardrum) by which sound waves reach the middle and inner ear.

AUDITORY CANAL-INTERNAL: The passage in the temporal bone petrous portion above the jugular foramen leading from the modiolus of the cochlea and ending as a horizontal shelf, the crista falciformis. It contains the facial (VII cranial) nerve, Auditory (VIII cranial) the cochlea and vestibular divisions, nervus intermedius (glossopalatine nerve) and basilar artery- internal auditory branch.

AUDITORY CAPSULE: In embryo development, the cartilaginous capsule which encloses the ear.

AUDITORY CENTER: The transverse temporal gyrus (area 41) below the Sylvius fissure of the temporal lobe, the auditory reception center.

AUDITORY CORTEX: The area of the outer layer of the brain, the terminal point for nerve impulses from the inner ear.

AUDITORY EMINENCE: Gray matter on the floor of the fourth ventricle on the brain.

AUDITORY FIELD: The distance, or space, within the limits of hearing.

AUDITORY GANGLION: (CORTI'S GANGLION) (SPIRAL GANGLION)
The collection of elongated nerve cells which pass from the modiolus to the organ of Corti.

AUDITORY MUSCLES: The stapedius and tensor tympani muscles of
the tympanic cavity (middle ear).

AUDITORY NERVE: (VESTIBULOCOCHLEARIS NERVE) VIII cranial,
a sensory nerve with two divisions. The cochlear division for au-
functioning has its origin in the spiral ganglion of the internal
auditory canal directed to the medulla. The vestibular division, for
body equilibrium has its origin from the cells of the vestibular
ganglion in the lateral end of the internal auditory canal, directed
to and entering the medulla oblongata. The branches are directed to
the semicircular ducts, saccule and utricle of the inner ear.

AUDITORY OSSICLES: The three small bones of the tympanic cavity
(middle ear), the malleus (hammer), incus (anvil) and stapes
(stirrup) which transmit sound waves from the tympanic membrane
(eardrum) to the fenestra vestibuli (oval window).

AUDITORY PLATE: The roof of the external auditory canal consisting
of bone.

AUDITORY RADIATION: A fiber tract from the medial geniculate nucleus to the temporal lobe transverse temporal gyrus (area 41).

AUDITORY RECEPTOR: A hair cell in the cochlea of the inner ear.

AUDITORY TEETH: (HUSCHK'S AUDITORY TEETH) Tiny toothlike projections on the vestibular, or inner edge, of the organ of Corti.

AUDITORY TUBE: (EUSTACHIAN TUBE) (TUBA PHARYNGOTYMPANICA)
Bartolomno Eustachio, Italian Anatomist. A canal from the tympanic cavity (middle ear) by which it communicates with the nasal
portion of the pharynx. It is lined with mucous membrane and
formed from bone, cartilage and fibrous tissue divided into the
cartilaginous, ishmus, membranous and osseous portions. It
provides for equalization of air pressure between the middle ear and
outside air   without rupture to the tympanic membrane (eardrum) and allows drainage of normal and diseased secretions from
the middle ear into the nasopharynx.

AURICLE: (AURICULA) (PINNA) The portion of the external ear

which protudes from the sides of the head. It surrounds the opening of the external auditory canal. It is formed from cartilage which is continuous with the external auditory canal and functions to collect and direct sound waves toward the middle and inner ear.

AURICULA CARTILAGE: A single piece of cartilage giving the external ear its framework and shape.

AURICULAR FISSURE: (TYMPANOMASTOIDEA FISSURE) A groove in the temporal bone petrous portion between the mastoid and tympanic portions.

AURICULAR LIGAMENTS: (VALSALVA'S LIGAMENTS) Antonio M. Valsalva, Italian Physician. The anterior, posterior and superior ligaments which assist in the attachment of the external ear to the side of the head.

AURICULARIS ANTERIOR MUSCLE: An extrinsic, thin muscle of the external ear. ORIGIN- The superficial fascia of the temporal area. INSERTION- The cartilage projection on the front of the helix. ACTION- Draws external ear forward and upward. NERVE- Facial (VII cranial) Temporal branch.

AURICULARIS POSTERIOR MUSCLE: A small bundle of extrinic fib - ers. ORIGIN- Temporal bone mastoid process. INSERTION- Inferior portion of the concha caranial surface. ACTION- Draws external ear backward. NERVE- Facial (VII cranial) posterior auricular branch.

AURICULARIS SUPERIOR MUSCLE: A fanshaped extrinic muscle of the external ear. ORIGIN- Superficial fasia of the temporal area. INSERTION- Superior cranial surface of the external ear. NERVE- Facial (VII cranial) temporal branch

AURICULOTEMPORAL NERVE: A sensory branch of the mandibular nerve, the third and largest division of the trigeminal (V cranial) nerve which further divides into: anterior auricular branches directed to the external ear helix and tragus; articular branches directed to the temporomandible joint; external acoustic meatus directed to the skin of the external auditory canal; parotid branches directed to the parotid gland; and superficial temporal branches directed to the skin of the temporal portion of the skull.

AURIFORM: Ear-shaped.

AURISCOPE: (MYRINGOSCOPE) (OTOSCOPE) Instrument for visual examination of the external auditory canal and tympanic membrane (eardrum).

AUTONOMIC: A portion of the nervous system uncontrolled by the brain or spinal cord. 2. Self controlling structure or system.

AUTONOMIC NERVE FIBERS: Fibers which are not under direct control, but controlled by neurons within the central nervous system. They are involved with such processes as the blood vessels, glands and the viscera.

AUTONOMIC NERVOUS SYTEM: (EFFERENT NERVOUS SYSTEM) (INVOLUNTARY NERVOUS SYSTEM) A division of the nervous system, an efferent (motor) system with fibers divided into two divisions. The parasympathic (craniosacral) division containing visceral efferent fibers which originate from the medulla and sacral portion of the spinal cord and the sympathetic (thoracolumbar) division receiving visceral fibers from a chain of fibers of the cell ganglia, one on each side of the spinal cord. The parasympathic division is associated with regulation processes and body maintenance and repair during the state of body rest. The sympathic division takes precedence and is dominant in emergency and stress situations by acceleration of heart beat, shutting off body activities such as digestion and diverting the blood supply to the peripheral muscular system for the fight or flight response.

AXIAL SKELETON: The skeleton of the head and trunk consisting of the hyoid bone, ribs, skull and vertebral column.

AXILLA: (ARMPIT) The small hollow under the arm. pl. axillae.

AXILLARY: Pertaining to, or located near, the armpit.

AXIS: The second cervical vertebra. 2. Imaginary line passing through the center of a body. 3. Line about which a rotating body turns.

AXON: (AXON CYLINDER) A process of a neuron which conducts impulses away from the cell body. It terminates in a synapse in the cent4al nervous system, ganglia or motor neuron. The axon with its sheath is a nerve fiber.

AXON HILLOCK: A conical elevation on a cell body of a neuron where the axon arises.

AZYGOS: To be one or unpaired.

B

BACCIFORM: Berry-shaped.

BACK: The functional portion of the tongue under the soft palate. 2. The posterior portion of the body from the neck down to the pelvis.

BACKBONE: (SPINE) (VERTEBRAL COLUMN) The portion of the axial skelton, from the coccyx to the cranium, consisting of the coccyx, sacrum and five lumbar, twelve thoracic and seven cervical verte- bra enclosing and protecting the spinal cord.

BALANCE ORGANS: The saccule, and the three semicircular canals, in three planes, and the utricle all located in the inner ear. The canals are along with the saccule and utricle all filled with endo- lymph fluid that moves in response to head movement. The fluid activate sensory hair cells which conduct impulses along the vest- ibular nerve, a division of the auditory (VIII cranial) nerve to the brain for orientation of body equilibrium.

BALL AND SOCKET JOINT: (ENARTHROSIS) A type of diarthrodial joint where the round end of one bone fits into the cavity of another. Allows angular and pivot movements in all directions.

BALLISTICS: Movements which result from sudden contractions and are continued by the inertia forces.

BAROMETER: Instrument for measuring atmospheric pressure. 2. Anything that marks change.

BASAL BODIES: A thickening at the base of each hairlike process attached to a free surface of a cell.

BASAL GANGLIA: Located under the third ventricle, it represents the gray matter and the thalamus in the middle of the cerebral hemi- sphere. It consist of the amygdaloid body, claustrum and corpus stria- tum; which consist of the caudate and lentiform nuclei and internal capsule.

BASAL PLATE: (BASALIS LAMINA) In embryo development, the lon- gitudinal zones of the nural tube ventral to the sulcus limitans. The gray columns of the spinal cord and the motor centers of the brain are formed from these zones.

BASE: (ROOT) The portion of the tongue connected with the hyoid bone by the hyoglossal membrane and genioglossus and hyoglossus muscles, and to the epiglottis by the glossoepiglottic mucous membrane; Also the soft palate by the glossopalatine arches and by mucous membrane and the constrictor pharyngis superior muscle.

BASEMENT MEMBRANE: A delicate noncellular structure under a layer of cells for attachment or support.

BASILAR ANGLE: The point formed by the intersection of a line from the nasal point, to a line drawn at the base of the nasal spine.

BASILAR ARTERY-INTERNAL AUDITORY: (COCHLEAR ARTERY) (LABYRINTHINE ARTERY) A branch from the basilar artery directed through the internal auditory canal of the inner ear.

BASILAR CREST: (CRISTA BASILARIS) A prominence projecting inward, and triangular in shape, from the spiral ligament to which is attached the basilar membrane of the organ of Corti.

BASILAR MACULAR: In embryo development, a cell cluster which developes into the basilar membrane of the organ of Corti.

BASILAR MEMBRANE: A membrane in the cochlea of the inner ear composed of transverse fibers that are directed perpendicular to the axis of the cochlea duct, embeded in a celleous substance. The tympanic surface is covered by a layer of skin containing vascular tissue. The width of the membrane is irregular and increases from the base, reaches maximum width at the end of the second turn, and then decreases sharply at the apex. It extends from the basilar crest to the tympanic lip of the spiral lamina, consisting of the zona arcuata, the inner portion on which the organ of Corti is supported, and the zona pectinata the outer portion.

BASILAR PART-OCCIPITAL BONE: A plate of bone joined to the sphenoid bone by cartilage, which ossifies with age forming one bone from the sphenoid and occipital bones.

BASILAR PORTION-OCCIPITAL BONE: (PARS BASILARIS) A quadrilateral portion of the occipital bone projecting forward and upward from the occipital bone magnum foramen, articulating with the sphenoid bone.

BASISPHENOID: The back portion of the sphenoid bone.

BELEMNOID: Dart-shaped.

BELL'S LAW: Charles Cell, Scottish Physiologist. Proposes that spinal nerve anterior roots contain motor fibers and the posterior roots contain sensory fibers.

BELLY: (VENTER) The fleshy portion of a muscle. 2. The stomach.

BEL: The measurement of acoustic or electrical power logarithm to base 10 of the power ratio: ten decibels.

BELONOID: Needle-shaped.

BERNOULLI EFFECT: J. Bernoulli, Swiss Mathematician. An aero-dynamic law which proposes; as velocity of fluid flow increases, pressure must decrease if the total energy remains constant. Pressure is perpendicular to the fluid flow direction; hence, velocity will increase at an area of constriction if volume fluid flow is constant, with a equal decrease in pressure at the constriction. This law is applied to phonation by assuming the vocal folds are closely together at the instant air is released by exhalation. The air stream will have a constant velocity until reaching the glottal constriction. As the air passes through the glottis the velocity will increase. A negative pressure results between the medial edges of the vocal folds, and they are therefore sucked toward each other (or midline).

BETA NERVE FIBERS: (GROUP B FIBERS) Fibers of the autonomic nervous system with a conduction speed of approximately 4. 5 meters per second.

BETWEEN BRAIN: (DIENCEPHALON) The second portion of the brain between the mesencephalon and telencephalon consisting of the epithalamus, hypothalamus, metathalamus and thalamus. Together with the telencephalon it forms the prosencephalon.

BETZ'S CELLS: (GIANT PYRAMIDAL CELLS) Vladimir A. Betz, Russian Anatomist. Large pyramidal ganglion cells forming layer V of the cerebral cortex's six cell layers.

BICUSPID: Having two cusps.

BICUSPID TOOTH: A tooth above and below on each side between the canines and molars.

BIFID: Divided into two parts.

BIFURCATION: To divide into two branches or parts.

BILABIAL: A consonant classification of articulators used, and the position they are in. With two lips.

BILATERAL: Pertaining to both sides.

BINAURAL: Pertaining to both ears.

BIPOLAR: Having two poles or processes.

BIPOLAR CELL: A neuron having two processes, a axon and a dendrite. These are found in the cochlea and the vestibular ganglia of the acoustic (VIII cranial) nerve.

BLADE: The functional portion of the tongue behind the tip and below the upper alveolar ridge. 2. A flat wide structure.

BLANDIN'S GLANDS: Phillippe F. BLANDIN,French Surgeon. The mucous and serous glands near the tip of the tongue.

BLAST: An immature, primitive cell.

BLASTOCOELE: In embryo development, the fluid filled cavity of the cell mass produced by attachment of a fertile egg.

BLASTOCYST: In embryo development, an outer layer to which is attached the inner mass of cells forming the blastocele cavity.

BLASTOMERE: In embryo development, a cell resulting from the clevage of a fertilized ovum.

BLASTOPHORE: The portion of a sperm cell not converted into sperm.

BLASTOPORE: In embryo development, the opening made by the blastula into the exterior of the embryo.

BLASTULA: A hollow ball of cells, one cell layer thick. pl. blastulae.

BODY CAVITIES: The four primary cavities are; peritoneal cavity in the abdomen; pericardial cavity containg the heart; and the two pleural cavities containing the lungs.

BODY CELL: A portion of a nerve cell, or neuron, which contains the nucleus and cytoplasm.

BODY-MAXILLA BONE: A somewhat pyramid-shaped bone, it contains the maxillary sinus cavity and has four surfaces; anterior, medial (nasal), posterior (infratemporal) and superior (orbital).

BODY PLANES: (ANATOMICAL PLANES) The three planes of the body; coronal (frontal), sagittal and transverse (horizontal).

PLANE	DIRECTION OF PLANE	DIVIDING INTO
Coronal (frontal)	Side-to-Side (lateral)	Front and Back parts
Sagittal	Front-to-Back	Right and Left parts
Transverse (horizontal	Horizontal (across)	Up)er and Lower parts

BODY-SPHENOID BONE: The center, cubical shaped, portion con-taining the sphenoidal air sinuses which are seperated at midline by a thin septrum.

BODY STALK: In embryo development, a band of mesoderm connect-ing the caudal end of the embryo with the chorion.

BODY SYSTEM: Two or more organs acting in combined functional unity.

SYSTEM	COMPOSED OF	SYSTEM STUDY
Articular	Joints and ligaments	Arthrology
Digestive	Digestive tract and digestive glands	Splanchnology
Endocrine	Ductless glands	-
Integument	Hair,nails and skin	Dermatology
Muscular	Flest portion, acting on the Articular and Skeletal systems	Myology
Nervous	Brain, ganglia, sense organs, spinal cord and associated nerves	Neurology
Reproductive	Organs of reproduction	-
Respiratory	Air passages and lungs	-
Skeletal	Bones and related cartilage	Osteology
Vascular	Blood vessels, heart and lymph	-

BOLUS: A rounded mass. 2. Pill shaped. 3. A soft mass of food.

BONE: A special type of connective tissue through which, due to its intercellular composition, rigidity is made possible. The intercell-ular composition is impregnated with mineral sale, calcium car-bonate, and calcium phosphate and containing approximately fifty percent solids and fifty percent water. Bone is classified as either compact or cancellous. Compact bone appears white and smooth. Cancellous bone appears porous. The major characreristic of bone is the lamellae (fibers and ground substance in layers). A canal system, the Haversian canals contains blood vessels and nerves. These canals are covered by concentric lamellae. Bone cells are within the oval-shaped lacunae (gaps or hollow spaces) within the lamellae. Smaller channels (canaliculi) extend out from the lacunae to communicate with the canaliculi of adjacent lacunae. Two types of bone marrow are contained with the network of cancellous bone. Red, manufacturing red blood cells and yellow which is adipose tissue. Periosteum, a tough fibrous membrane covers the outside of bone. The inner layer contains osteoblasts cells responsible for bone formation. Bone shapes are classified as; Flat-in the cranium. Long-in the arms and legs. Irregular and Short- in the feet, hands, and vertebrae.

BONE CELL: Consists of a flat, nucleated, cell, each one in a seperate small hollow space in bone.

BONE CONDUCTION: The process of sound conduction through the cranial bones directed to the cochlea of the inner ear.

BONE MARROW: (MARROW) The soft material filling the cavities of spongy bone. It consist of red marrow which produces red blood cells and is found in flat and short bones such as ribs, sternum and vertebrae bodies. Yellow marrow, which is fat cells is found in the large cavities of long bones in the arms and legs.

BONY COCHLEA: The cavity within the petrous portion of the temporal bone which contains the cochlea.

BONY LABYRINTH: (OSSEOUS LABYRINTH) The cavities of the inner ear in the temporal bone petrous portion lined with periosteum and containing perilymph fluid. These cavities consists of the cochlea, semicircular canals and vestibule.

BORDER: The outer edge or boundry line.

BOYLE'S LAW: Robert Boyle, British Physicist. Proposes that the volume of a given mass of gas at a constant temperature is inversely proportional to one another and produce a constant product. Expressed as: (pressure) x (volume)   constant (at a constant temp - erature)

BRAIN: The large organ of soft nerve tissue of the central nervous system within the cranium including neural and thought coordin- ation and higher nerve centers which receive stimuli from the sense organs and correlating of stimuli to form motor impulses. It consist of neurons and nutritives and the cerebrum, cerebellum, medulla oblongata, midbrain and pons.

BRAIN STEM: Consist of the diencephalon, medulla, midbrain and pons.

BRANCHIAL ARCHES: (PHARYNGEAL POUCHES) (VISCERAL ARCHES) In embryo development, five pair of arches from which face and neck structures are formed. The mandibular, or first arch, forms the anterior portion of the tongue, lower lip, mandible bone and muscles of mastication. The hyoid or second arch, forms the hyoid bone lesser cornu, stapes, styoid process and stylohyoid ligament. The third arch forms the hyoid bone greater cornu and the posterior portion of the tongue. The fourth arch forms the thyroid cartilage and from the fifth arch the arytenoid and cricoid cartilages are formed.

BRANCHIAL CLEFTS: In embryo development, the opening between the branchial arches.

BRANCHIAL GROOVES: (GILL CLEFTS) In embryo development, a number of slight furrows which seperate the branchial arches.

BRANCHIAL MUSCLES: In embryo development, most of the muscles of the face and neck developed from the mesoderm of the arches.

BRANCHIAL PLEXUS:The lower cervical nerves and dorsal spine nerves directed to the aur, forearm and hand.

BRACHIUM: A armlike process or structure.

BRACHIUM PONTIS: (MIDDLE CEREBELLAR PEDUNCLE) An area of the internal cerebellum which contains, on each side, fibers of the pons.

BRACHIUM CONJUNCTIVUM: (SUPERIOR CEREBELLAR PEDUNCLE) The lateral wall on each side of the cephalic portion of the fourth ventricle.

BREAST BONE: (STERNUM BONE) A flat oblong bone in the midline at the front of the thorax. In the front it forms the anterior wall of the thorax, and joined above with the clavicle bones, and on the lateral surface by seven pair of indentations, for articulation of the costal cartilage of the seven pair of true ribs. The lowest portion, the xiphoid (ensiform) process, has no ribs attached but some abdominal muscle are attached.

BREATHING: Process of inflating and deflating the lungs for carbon dioxide for oxygen exchange.

BREATHING CYCLE: At rest, envirement and pressure within the lungs is the same. With the initiating of breathing, the anterior muscle fibers draw the central tendon down and forward, and the posterior fibers contract to increase the vertical diameter of the thorax. The intercostal muscles cause the ribs to turn outward and enlarge on the anterior, lateral, and posterior diameters of the thorax. The size increase results in negative pressure in the lungs verses the envirement and air rushes in until the pressure is equalized. The downward and forward motion of diaphragm exerts pressure on the abdomen and raises the internal abdominal pres - sureThe forces of gravity, tissue elasticity and torque return the thorax to the position of rest and the intraoulmonic pressure is raised. Air is exhaled from the lungs until the intrapulmonic pres- sure is again equal to the envirement.

BREATHY: (ASTHENIC: Vocal quality due to the incomplete blockage of the air passage. It is most noticeable at the beginning of the ex- piratory cycle and limits the range of intensity due to organically caused, or poor vocal habits.

BRIDGE: (PONS) A swelling of fibers on the brain stem ventral sur- face between the midbrain cerebral peduncles and medulla oblongata. It contains fiber tracts and from its border the abducent (XI cranial) auditory (VIII cranial), facial (VII cranial) and trigeminal (V cra- inal) nerves have their origin.

BRIDGE OF THE NOSE: (NASAL BONES) Two small oblong bones lo- cater´ side by side at point of midline and superior portion of the face. They articulate with the frontal bone and the ethmoid bone perpendicular plate.

BROCA'S AREA: (AREA 44-45) (SPEECH CENTER) Pierre P. Broca, French Surgeon. The area on the left side of the brain in the inferior frontal gyrus rostal to the motor area (area 8) for motor speech.

BROCA'S CONVOLUTION: The inferior frontal gyrus, area 44-45.

BROCA'S FISSURE: The fissure which encircles the inferior frontal gyrus.

BRONCHI: The main branch leading from the trachea provides the passage way for air moving from and to the lungs. It bifurcates (divides) opposite the third thoracic vertebra. At this point any foreign matter too large to enter either bronchus would rest after passing through the trachea. The division forms the left and right bronchi, each slightly more than half the diameter of the trachea. The right bronchus is shorter and more vertical than the left. They enter the lungs and terminate in the bronchioles, or bronchial tubes. They are composed of cartilaginous rings connected by fibroelastic tissue. The left bronchus divides into two secondary bronchi which further subdivide into eight third order bronchi which supply each lung segment. The right bronchus divides into three secondary bronchi one for each lobe of the lung. The secondary bronchi further subdivides into ten third order bronchi which each supply a lung segment.

BRONCHIOLE: A small final subdivision of the third order bronchi. The bronchi   further subdive until they end in terminal bronchioles that lack cartilage, and communicate with alvolar ducts that open into the lung air sacs. pl. bronchioli.

BRONCHUS: One of the two large branches of the trachea for air passage to the lungs. pl. bronchi.

BROWNIAN MOTION: (BROWNIAN MOVEMENT) Robert Brown, English Botanist. The rapid, random, movement of microscopic particles suspended in gases or liquids.

BUCCAE: (CHEEKS) Forming the sides of the face; the external portion being skin, the internal portion mucous membrane. Between the layers are fat, facial muscles, glands and mastication muscles.

BUCCAL CAVITY: (MOUTH CAVITY) Consists of the vestibule, with external boundries of the cheeks and lips and mouth cavity proper with internal boundries of the gingivae (gums) and teeth. Its shape and size depend on the structure of the cheeks and lips.

BUCCAL FAT PAD: (PAD OF BICHAT) (SUCTORIAL PAD) Marie F. Bichat, French Anatomist. A deposit of fat in the cheeks superficial to the buccinator muscle. This pad is prominent in infants and assists in the sucking action.

BUCCAL NERVE: A sensory branch of the mandibular nerve, the third and largest division of the trigeminal (V cranial) nerve directed to portions of the cheeks,gingivae (gums) and mouth.

BUCCAL NERVE BRANCHES: Motor branch of the facial (VII cranial) nerve directed to the buccinator and orbicularis oris muscles, small muscles of the nose and superficial muscles of the face.

BUCCAL GLANDS: Small glands in the mucous membranes of the mouth which secrete saliva.

BUCCINATOR MUSCLE: The deepest of the facial muscles, and major muscle of the cheek. ORIGIN-Maxilla bone alveolar process; mandible bone ridge. DIRECTION- Horizontal and medial. INSERTION- Orbicularis oris muscle at mouth angle. ACTION- Compresses cheek, retracts angle of mouth. NERVE- Facial (VII cranial) buccal branch.

BUCCONASAL MEMBRANE: In embryo development, a epithelial membrane which closes the end of each olfactory pit. When the membranes rupture the primitive choanae (openings) are made.

BUCCOPHARNGEAL MEMBRANE: (ORAL PLATE) In embryo development, the plate forming the seperation between the foregut and oral groove; also the location for the opening into the mouth.

BUCCULA: (DOUBLE CHIN) A fold of fatty tissue under the chin.

BUCK: (TRAGUS) Gordon Buck, American Surgeon. A small tongue like cartilaginous projection in front of the outer ear external canal.

BULBIFORM: Bulb-shaped.

BULK MODULUS OF ELASTICITY: (VOLUME MODULUS OF ELASTICITY) When compressional forces act inward over a surface area, the volume is compressed. The co-efficient of compression is the bulk modulus of elasticity. It is determined by the restoring force of the compressed substance.

BUNDLE OF RASMUSSEN: (OLIVOCOCHLEA BUNDLE) G;L; Rasmussen. A bundle of efferent nerve fibers between the cochlea and olivary complex.

BURDACH'S FISSURE: Karl F. Burdach, German Physiologist. A fissure between the inner surface of the operculum and lateral surface of the insula.

BURSA: A sac or saclike cavity. 2. A sac or cavity containing synovia fluid which reduces the friction between bone and tendon or ligament and tendon.

BUTTOCKS: The rounded part of either side of the lower back that forms the rump or seat.

C

CALCARINE SULCUS: Located on the occipital lobe, medial surface, between the cuneus and lingual gyrus.

CALCIUM CARBONATE-OF LIME: The otocnium or ear dust of the inner ear saccule and utricle.

CALLOSOMARGINAL FISSURE: (CINGULI SULCUS) Located on the medial surface of a cerebral hemisphere and seperates the cingulate gyrus from the paracentral lobe and superior frontal gyrus.

CANAL: A narrow channel or passage.

CANAL OF HUGUIER: (ITER CHORDAE ANTERIUS) Pierre C. Huguier, French Surgeon. A canal through which the chorda tympani nerve exits into the tympanic cavity (middle ear).

CANAL REUNIENS: (DUCT OF HENSEN) (REUNIENS DUCT) A membranous short tube from the scala media (cochlea duct) to the saccula in the vestibule of the inner ear which allows endolymph fluid interchange.

CANAL OF ROSENTHAL: (SPIRAL CANAL OF THE MODIOLUS) Isidor Rosenthal, German Physiologist. A passage containing the spiral ganglion of the cochlear division of the auditory (VIII cranial) nerve which follows the direction of the osseous spiral lamina of the inner ear.

CANALICULUS: Very small tube shaped channel or passage. 2. a number of small channels or passages. pl. canaliculi.

CANCELLOUS BONE: (SPONGY BONE) Bone substance of thin, intersecting lamellae, of bars and plates, forming many communicating spaces filled with bone marrow in the interior of a bone.

CANINE: A canine tooth or pertaining to the canine teeth.

CANINE EMINENCE: A bony ridge overlying the root of the canine tooth on both the mandible and maxilla bones.

CANINE FOSSA: A wide depression on the anterior surface of the maxilla bone, lateral to the incisive fossa and supralateral to the canine tooth socket.

CANINE MUSCLE: (LEVATOR ANGULI ORIS) A muscle of the mouth for facial expression. ORIGIN- Maxilla bone canine fossa. DIREC-TION- Downward and oblique. INSERTION- Orbicularis oris muscle and the skin at the mouth angle. ACTION- Raises mouth angle. NERVE- Facial (VII cranial) .

CANINE TEETH: (EYE TEETH) The four teeth, one on either side of each jaw, between the incisors and molars with a cone-shaped crown and a single root; used for tearing. Approximate eruption: Deciduous 18-24 months, Permanent 12-14 years.

CAPILLARY: The smallest vessel of the vascular system. Aids in conducting blood from arteries to veins.

CAPITULUM: A small protrusion on a bone that articulates with an-other bone. pl. capitula

CAPSULE: A membrane acting as a container.

CARBON DIOXIDE Acolorless, odorless, gas heavier than air, formed in body tissue and expelled by the lungs. Symbol: CO_2

CARDIAC: Pertaining to the heart. 2. A person with a heart disorder.

CARDIAC MUSCLE: Found only in the heart, being both smooth and striated muscle. Composed of a majority of fibrous connective tissue.

CARDINAL VOWELS: (VOWELS) A system of sounds with perceptual quality the same, regardless of the spoken language, that are des-criptive of the physiological limits of the tongue positions for the vowel sounds.

CARIES: Molecular decay of bone. It becomes discolored, porous and soft producing a chronic inflammation of the surrounding tissue.

CARNIVOROUS: Flesh eating.

CAROTID: Artery directed from the neck to the brain.

CAROTID CANAL: A canal in the temporal bone petrous portion di-rected vertically, bends and then horizontally forward and medial-ward. It communicates with the cranium, internal carotid artery and plexus of nerves.

CAROTID GROOVE: (CAROTID SULCUS) A wide groove on the side of the sphenoid bone body which contains the carotid artery and cavernous sinus.

CAROTID SINUS NERVE: A sensory branch of the glossopharyngeal (IX cranial) nerve directed to the carotid artery with blood pressure receptors.

CAROTID WALL: (ANTERIOR WALL) A wall of the tympanic cavity (middle ear) that is wider at the top than the bottom. A thin plate of bone seperates it from the carotid canal. The top portion of the wall is perforated by a tendon for the tensor tympani muscle and the opening of the auditory (eustachian) tube. They are seperated by a thin horizontal plate of bone: the sepum canalis musculotubarii.

CARTILAGE: A type of dense connective tissue. It's composition of cells, ground substance and intercellular fibers give it firmness, yet some elasticity. This composition renders it capable of withstanding much pressure and tension. It is found in the bronchi; between the vertebra bodies; costal cartilages of the ribs; covering the articular surface of bone; external ear; auditory tube lining; nasal septum; trachea; and the wall of the larynx. By its nature of fibrous substance, it is divided into three types, elastic, fibrous and hyline.

CARTILAGES OF SANTORINI: (CORNICULATE CARTILAGES) Giovamni D. Santorini, Italian anatomist. The apex of each arytenoid cartilage is pointed, curved backward and medial, topped with a conical cartilaginous nodule; the corniculate cartilage. Each nodule consist of elastic cartilage, articulating with the tops of the arytenoid cartilage. They are located in the posterior portion of the aryepiglottic folds of mucous membrane.

CARTILAGINOUS GLOTTIS: The posterior portion of the rima glottis; bounded by the vocal processes and the medial surfaces of the arytenoid cartilages.

CARTILAGINOUS PORTION-AUDITORY TUBE) A plate of elastic cartilage formed into a triangle. The top portion attaches to the osseous portion of the tube, and the base attaches under the mucous membrane of the nasal part of the pharynx forming an elevation: torus tubarius (cushion); behind the orifice of the tube. The top edge is curled upon itself to present the appearance of a hook when viewed in transverse.

CATHETER: Tube that is passed into body passages, often for drawing off fluid.

CATHODE: The negative (-) pole, the opposite of the anode, or positive (+) pole.

CATION: The element of an electrolyte in electrochemical decomposition at the cathode, or negative (-) pole, appearing as a positive (+) ion.

CAUDA: Shaped like a tail. 2. A tail-like appendage. pl. caudae.

CAUDA EQUINA: The collection of roots and lower spinal nerves below the termination of the spinal cord.

CAUDA HELICIS: A pointed porcess which extends inferiorly from the helix of the external ear.

CAUDAL: Away from the head, toward the tail.

CAUDATE NUCLEUS: A prominent portion of the lateral medial ventricle curved forming an arch. The head is enlarged contained by the lateral wall with the tail portion seperated from the thalamus by the stria terminalis.

CAVE: The small area ouside the external canal on the external ear.

CAVERNOUS: Containing hollow spaces.

CAVERNOUS SINUS: A irregular space between the sphenoid bone body from the fissure to the apex of the temporal bone petrous portion.

CAVITY: Hollow, or space, within or between structures.

CAVITY TONE THEORY: Proposes that the vowel sounds are dependent on the resonating tube length. By increasing the length the vowels are produced in the following order; i, e, a, o, u.

CAVUM TYMPANI: The tympanic cavity or middle ear.

CECUM: A cavity closed at one end or a cul-de-sac.

CELL: The physiological and structural unit of the body. They differ in size and shape. The average diameter of a red blood cell is about 0.0075 millimeter and approximately one fourth as thick. A striated muscle may be an inch or more long but the diameter is usually less than 0. 05 millimeters. The major portions of a cell include the; cellular membrane, cytoplasm, golgi apparatus, centrophere, and nucleus.

CELLS OF CLAUDIUS: Friedrich Claudius, Austrian Anatomist. The large columnar supporting cells on the basilar membrane, external to the organ of Corti. The cells are secretory, and with vascular tissue form the stri vascularis, which secrete endolumph fluid in the inner ear.

CELLS OF DEITER: Otto Deiter, German Anatomist. The supporting phalanges (finger-like) cells with their base resting on the basilar membrane, with club-like processes interspersed among the outer hair cells of the organ of Corti.

CELLS OF MARTINOTTI: Giouanni Martinotti, Bologna Pathologist. Spindle-shaped cells with long processes located in the polymorphic layer (Layer VI) of the cerebral cortex.

CELLULAR MEMBRANE: The thin capsule surrounding a cell. Its membrane contains lipide, protein molecules and tiny holes or pores. These pores are few in each cell. The cellular membrane prevents the leakage of inner cellular structures into the surrounding environment. It serves as a selective barrier keeping unwanted substances from entering the cell, and admitting other substances that are required for maintaining cell life.

CEMENTUM: A layer of bony material on the dentine of the tooth root.

CENTER: The middle point of the body. A group of nerve cells responsible for a specific function.

CENTRAL CANAL: A small canal in the center of the spinal cord extending its full length directed to the apex into medulla oblongata. Opening into the fourth ventricle and lined with ependyma cells, it contains cerebrospinal fluid.

CENTRAL LOBE: (ISLAND OF REIL) (INSULA) A triangular shaped area in the cerebral cortex forming the floor of the lateral cerebral fossa. pl. insulae.

CENTRAL NERVOUS SYSTEM: Consists of the brain and spinal cord controlling voluntary actions. This includes portions of the brain controlling consciousness and mental activity, the spinal cord and their motor and sensory nerve fibers which control muscles. It is composed of tissue with both gray and white matter, the gray matter being composed of cells of nervous tissue and the white matter composed of nerve fibers from the cells. Impulses are carried from the body by the white matter in the brain and spinal cord.

CENTRAL SULCUS: (FISSURE OF ROLANDO) Divides the frontal and parietal lobes of each cerebral hemisphere. It begins at approximately midline between the inferior and superior borders and is directed up and backward to its termination near the midline of the superior border.

CENTRAL TENDON: A strong, thin uneven sheet of tendon, trileaf-shaped in the diaphragm. It consists of several layers of fibers which intersect at angles giving strength with little elasticity to it. The muscular portion consist of the costal, sternal and vertebral processes.

CENTRAL TENDON-MUSCULAR PROCESS:
    COSTAL PORTION:
        ORIGIN- Lower border and inner surfaces of the cartilages of ribs senve through twelve. DIRECTION- Upward and medial. INSERTION- Central tendon. NERVE-Phrenic from cervical plexus.
    STERNAL PORTION:
        ORIGIN- Lower border and back of the sternum eniform process. DIRECTION- Upward and medial. INSERTION- Front of middle leaf of the central tendon. NERVE- Phrenic from cervical plexus.
    VERTEBRAL PORTION: Origin from two crus of muscle fiber.
        ORIGIN- LEFT CRUS- From the two upper lumbar vertebrae and interventebral disk. DIRECTION- Vertical upward and medial. INSERTION- Central tendon. NERVE- Phrenic from cervical plexus.

        ORIGIN-RIGHT CRUS- From the upper three or four lumbar vertebrae and interventebral disk. DIRECTION- Upward, fanning out and medial. INSERTION- Crossing over and encircules the esophagus inserting into the central tendon.

CENTROSOME: (CENTROSPHERE) A spherical body located near the center of the cell, close to the nucleus. It is composed of a pair of rod-shaped granules and centrioles. The centrioles have a role in prophase, the first phase of cell division.

CEPHALAD: (CRANIAL) (ROSTRAD)Toward the head or superior portion of the body.

CEREBELLI VERMIS: The median portion of brain between the hemi-spheres.

CEREBELLUM: The largest portion of the hindbrain consisting of two lateral cerebellar hemispheres and the vermis, a narrow medial portion. It is connected to the brain by three pair of peduncles, the inferior with the medulla oblongata, middle with the pons and sup-erior with the cerebrum. Its major function is the co-ordination of voluntary muscular movements, receiving afferent impulses and sending efferent impulses.

CEREBELLUM TONSILLA: A round shaped mass forming a portion of the cerebellum on the inferior surface between the biventral lobe and the uvula.

CEREBRAL CORTEX: The convoluted layer of gray matter which cov-ers the hemispheres. Approximately is hidden from view in the sulci walls. The layers are dark and light formed by myelinated nerve fibers and nerve cell bodies. The cortex is divided into six layers. The outer plexiform layer (Layer I) is a narrow white layer containing the granular cells, horizontal cells, and the termina-tion point for dentrites of pyramidal cells. The external granular layer (Layer II) contains granule (Type II Golgi), and the shafts of the pyramidal and small pyramidal cells. The layer of pyramidal cells (Layer III) divides into portions, the inner portion with large pyramidal cells and the outer portion with medium size pyramidal cells. It contains the cells of Martinotti and stellate cells. The in-ternal granular layer (Layer IV) contains many small stellate cells and a few small pyramidal cells. It contains the synapses with layer III pyramidal cells. The ganglionic layer (Layer V) contains the layer of large pyramidal cells of Betz and the large pyrmidal cells. The polymorphic layer (Layer VI) contains irregular shaped cells whose axons penetrate the adjacent white matter of the hemisphere.

CEREBRAL PEDUNCLES: The ventral portion of the midbrain consisting of a pair of white bundles from the cerebrum to the superior portion of the pons.

39

CEREBROSPINAL FLUID: (SPINAL FLUID) A clear fluid covering the brain and spinal cord. The fluid is produced by highly vascular folds or processes (choroid plexuses) of the pia mater layer in the ventricles and functions as a fluid shock absorber and nutritive for nerve cells.

CEREBROSPINAL NERVE: A nerve with its origin in the brain or spinal cord.

CEREBRUM: A large portion of the brain, occupying the upper part of the cranium. It is divided incompletely into two major (right and left) hemispheres that contain many convolutions and fissures. The cerebrum functions in the interpretation of sensation, sensory impulses, and voluntary muscular actions. In addition it is the center for the mental activities of emotions, intelligence, judgement, learning and memory.

CEREBRUM AQUEDUCT: (AQUEDUCT OF SYLVIUS) Jacobus Sylvius, French Anatomist. A narrow canal from the third to the fourth ventricle of the brain through which cerebrospinal fluid passes.

CEREBRUM FISSURES: The five major fissures are; longitudinal, which seperates the two hemispheres: transverse, between the cerebellum and the cerebrum, central sulcus (fissure of Rolando), lateral (fissure of Sylvius) and parieto-occipital.

CEREBRUM LOBE: Each hemisphere is divided into four lobes;as the cranial bones, frontal, occipital, parietal, and temporal.

CERUMEN: (EAR WAX) A soft secretion found only in the external auditory canal. It serves as a protective device for self cleansing of the ear.

CERUMINOUS GLANDS: Located in the external auditory canal; for secreting cerumen (earwax)

CERVICAL: Pertaining to the neck or nerves.

CERVICAL GANGLION; A portion of the sympathetic trunk consisting of the inferior, middle and superior ganglion.

CERVICAL NERVE BRANCH: A motor branch of the facial (VII cranial) nerve directed to the platysma muscle.

CERVICAL PLEXUS: Nerve plexus formed by the ventral divisions of the superior four cervical nerves; serves to communicate to the facial and anterior neck regions.

CERVICAL SINUS: In embryo development, the temporary structure formed by the disappearance of the third and fourth branchial arch-ea. Located between the thoracic wall from behind and in the hyoid arch in front.

CERVICAL VERTEBRA: The first seven bones of the spinal column.

CERVIX: Neck of a organ or structure. 2. Lower front portion of the part connecting the head and trunk. pl. cervixes.

CESIUM: Alkali similar to potassium and sodium. Symbol- Cs.

CHAIN GANGLION: (TRUNK GANGLION) Nerve cell bodies in groups along the sympathetic trunk.

CHEEK BONE: (MALAR BONE) (ZYGOMATIC BONE) Located at the lateral and upper portion of the face. Quadrangular in shape with frontosphenoidal, maxillary, orbital and temporal processes and the malar (outer) and temporal surfaces. It forms, along with the zygomatic process of the maxilla and temporal bones, the zygomatic arch (cheek bone) and a portion of the orbital cavity lateral floor and wall. It articulates with the frontal, maxilla, spenoid and temporal bones.

CHEEKS: (BUCCAE) Forming the sides of the face; the external por-tion being skin, the internal portion mucous membrane. Between the layers are fat, facial muscles, glands and mastication muscles.

CHEMORECEPTOR: A sensory receptor which is highly specialized; stimulated by a body chemical substance as in a taste bud.

CHIASMA: Decussation, or X-shaped crossing of fibers; as in the optic chiasma.

CHIN: (MENTAL PROTUBERANCE) (POINT OF THE CHIN) A triangular projection formed by the dividing of the midline ridge (mental sym-physis) near the lower border of the mandible bone.

CHLORINE: A heavy, yellowish-green, gaseous element of irritating odor. Symbol, Cl.

CHOANA: Funnel shaped cavity. 2. the openings between the basal cavity and the nasopharynx. pl. choanae.

CHONDRAL: Pertaining to cartilage.

CHONDROCLAST: A large cell associated with the absorption of cartilage.

CHONDROGLOSSUS MUSCLE: A extrinsic muscle of the tongue considered to be a part of the Hyoglossus muscle. ORIGIN- Hyoid bone body and lesser cornu. DIRECTION- Upward. INSERTION- Between the genioglossus and hyoglossus muscles. ACTION- Depress and retract tongue. NERVE- Hypoglossal (XII cranial).

CHORDA: A cord or tendon. pl. chordae.

CHORDA TYMPANI NERVE: A sensory branch of the facial (VII cra - nial) nerve directed to the anterior two thirds of the tongue and the sublingual and submandibular glands.

CHORION: In embryo development, the external membrane enclosing the fertilized ovum, serving as a nutritive and protective covering.

CHORION FRONDOSUM: In embryo development, an area of the chorion where the villi, in contact with the decidua basalis, increase in size becoming the placenta fetal portion.

CHORIONIC VILLI: In embryo development, small, threadlike projections on the external surface of the chorion.

CHOROID: Similar to the chorion.

CHOROID PLEXUS: A vascular fold of the pia mater, in the superior portion of the lateral ventricle inferior horn, which assist in the production of cerebrospinal fluid.

CHROMATIDS: The two parts forming a chromosome which split in mitosis (cell division).

CHROMATOLYSIS: The disintegration, due to exhaustion, fatigue, or injury, on the Nissl bodies of a nerve cell.

CHROMOSOME: The rod-like (J or V shaped) body which appears in the nucleus of a cell at the time of mitosis (cell division). In man the number is constant, being twenty three pair.

CHRONAXIE TIME: (EXCITATION TIME) Time required for the excitation of a nervous element by a definite stimulus. 2. Minimum time at which current just doubles the rheobase and excite contraction.

CHRONIC: Long lasting.

CILIA: Hairlike processes projecting from epithelial cells which move dust, mucous or pus.

CILIARY GANGLION: [CILIARY ROOT) A sensory ganglion from the nasociliary nerve, a branch of the ophthalmic nerve, the first division of the trigeminal (V cranial) nerve directed along the optic (II cranial) nerve to the eye bulb.

CILIARY NERVES: Two small sensory nerves from the nasociliary nerve, a branch of the ophthalmic nerve, the first division of the trigeminal (V cranial) nerve directed to the eye cornea and iris.

CILIATED CELLS: Cells which have microscopic hairlike structures from the cell body. 2. Hair cells in the organ of Corti.

CILIUM: Thread-like cytoplasmic processes of cells which beat rhythmically. Located on cell borders and responsible for movement of food and wastes.

CINEFLUOROGRAPHY: X-ray radiography combined with motion-picture photography.

CINEMATOGRAPHY: Photography using motion pictures.

CINEREA: Gray matter of the nervous system.

CINGULATE GYRUS: A convolution in an arch-shape, near the surface of the callosal sulcus.

CINGULATE SULCUS: A long irregularly shaped, sulcus from the corpus callosum anterior limit, divided parallel and terminates behind the central sulcus.

CINGULI SULCUS: (CALLOSOMARGINAL FISSURE) Located on the medial surface of a cerebral hemisphere and seperates the cingulate gyrus from the paracentral lobe and superior frontal gyrus.

CINGULUM: A confining or encirculing structure.

CIRCUMDUCTION: Active or passive circular movement of a limb.

CIRCUMVALLATE PAPILLAE: The largest papillae on the tongue consisting of approximately eight to twelve arranged in a V shape.

Cl: Cymbol for chlorine. A heavy yellowish-green gaseous element of irritating odor.

CLAUSTRUM: A thin layer of gray matter outside the external capsule of the brain, dividing it from the white matter of the insula.

CLAVICLE BONE: (COLLAR BONE) A bone shaped like the letter f that articulates with the sternum and scapula bones. The head articulates with the manibrium of the sternum by arthrodial joints. The lateral end articulates with the acromion (hook-shaped projection) on the scapula.

CLAVICULAR NOTCH: The upper angle of the sternum bone with which the clavicle bone articulates.

CLEFT: A long fissure which divides or splits.

CO_2: Symbol for carbon dioxide.

COCCYGEAL NERVES: A pair of nerves arising from the coccyx portion of the spinal cord which enter the pudendal plexus.

COCCYX: The small bone at the base of the spinal column formed by three or four fused vertebrae. Articulation is by small intervertebral disk with the sacrum.

COCHLEA: The essential organ of hearing in the inner ear curled upon itself around a bony central axis, the modiolus in a snail-shape. The cochlea contains the organ of Corti; the end organ of hearing where sound waves are converted into nerve impulses. The spiral lamina, a bony plate extends from the modiolus and partially divides the cochlea into two portions; the scala tympani communicating with the fenestra rotunda (round window) and the scala vestibuli communicating with the fenestra vestibuli (oval window). Between the two is the scala media (cochlear duct containing the organ of Corti. The two scalae communicate at the apex through the helicotrema.

COCHLEA DUCT: (MEMBRANOUS COCHLEA) (SCALA MEDIA) The tube triangular shaped within the cochlea separated from the scala vestibuli by Reissner's membrane and from the scala tympani by the basilar membrane. The duct contains the organ of Corti and endolymph fluid.

COCHLEA PROCESS: A thin plate of bone separating the auditory (Eustachian) tube from the canal through which the tensor tympani muscle is directed to the malleus bone of the tympanic cavity (middle ear).

COCHLEA RECESS: A small depression between the fenestra vestibuli (oval window) and fenestra rotunda (round window) which forms the vestibular portion of the cochlea duct (scala media).

COCHLEA AQUEDUCT: A passage through which the perilymphatic and subarachnoid areas communicate.

COCHLEA ARTERY: (BASILAR ARTERY-INTERNAL AUDITORY) (LAB-YRINTHINE ARTERY) A branch from the basilar artery directed through the internal auditory canal of the inner ear.

COCHLEA MICROPHONICS: Minute quantities of electrical energy generated within the cochlea. The energy has properties analogous to thoses of acoustic stimulus.

COCHLEA NERVE: A division of the auditory (VIII cranial) nerve with its origin from the spiral ganglion of the cochlea. The fibers of the central portion are directed through the modiolus into the internal auditory canal directed to the cochlea nuclei. The peripheral fibers are directed to the organ of Corti.

COCHLEAR NUCLEUS: The terminal point of the cochlea nerve fibers from which the central auditory pathways arise.

COCHLEARIFORM: Spoon shaped.

COCHLEARIFORM PROCESS: A plate of bone above the fenestra vestibuli (oval window) which is spoon-shaped.

COELOM: In embryo development, the body cavity of the embryo between the lateral mesoderm layers.

COLLAR BONE: (CLAVICLE BONE) A bone shaped like the letter f which articulates with the sternum and scapula bones. The head articulates with the manibrium of the sternum by arthrodial joints. The lateral end articulates with the acromion (hook-shaped projection) on the scapula.

COLLATERAL: A tiny side branch of an axon or neuron.

COLLICULUS: Small elevation or mound. pl. colliculi.

COLUMELLA: A tiny column.

COLUMELLA COCHLEAE: The modiolus of the inner ear on which the cochlea is curled.

COLUMN: A pillar or supporting structure.

COLUMNAR CELL: A epithelial cell that has more height than width.

COMMISSURE: The joining site of corresponding parts.

COMPACT BONE: (DENSE BONE) Bone on the exterior portion of a bone containing fewer microscopic spaces, being dense and hard.

COMPLEMENTAL AIR: (INSPIRATORY RESERVE VOLUMN) The quantity of air which can be inhaled beyond that inhaled during quiet breathing.

COMPARTATIVE ANATOMY: Comparison of the anatomy of different orders of animals or plants, one with another.

COMPLEX TONE: A sound wave consisting of a number of pure tones.

COMPRESSION: The position of a sound wave when air particles are forced against each other. When the force is applied there is an increase in air pressure.

CONCAVE: A rounded depression, or hollow surface.

CONCHA: The shell-like, deepest cavity of the external ear in which is located the entrance to the external auditory canal. 2. One of the three nasal concha. pl. conchae.

CONCHAE AURICULAE CYMBA: The upper portion of the concha of the external ear.

CONDENSER LENS: Lens that concentrates light energy. A positive lens.

CONDYLE: A rounded, or knuckle-like, process. 2. A round protusion at bone ends.

CONDYLOID CANAL: A small channel in the occipital bone condyloid fossa for passage of the transverse sinus vein.

CONDYLOID FOSSA: The slight depression on each side of the occipital bone foramen magnum.

CONDYLOID JOINT: Type of diarthrodial joint which permits all angular movement except rotation. 2. Shaped like a knuckle.

CONDYLOID PROCESS-MANDIBLE BONE: An articulating process on the mandible bone ramus portion presenting a surface for articulation with the articular disk of the temporomandibular joint. The neck portion is convex on the posterior and the anterior containing a depression for the insertion of the external pterygoid muscle.

CONE OF LIGHT: An area on the tympanic membrane (eardrum), tri-angular in shape, which appears brighter than the rest of the membrane when viewed through an otoscope. It is the sign of a healthy eardrum and tympanic cavity (middle ear).

CONGENITAL: Existing at birth, may or may not be hereditary.

CONNECTIVE TISSUE: Serves to bind, connect, or support, other tissue and parts. The tissue has few cells in number and a large amount of intercellular substance and slightly vascular except for cartilage. It is subdivided by the intercellular substance into: connective tissue proper, adipose, areolar, dense fibrous, mucous and reticular. Dense connective tissue includes bone and cartilage.

CONSTRICTOR PHARYNGIS INFERIOR MUSCLE: (INFERIOR CON-STRICTOR MUSCLE) A strong, thick muscle of the pharynx. ORIGIN- From the sides of the cricoid and thyroid cartilage. DIRECTION- Backward and medial. INSERTION- On the medial raphe of the pos-terior wall of the pharynx. ACTION- Constricts the pharynx. NERVE- Vagus (X cranial) laryngeal external and recurrent nerve branches. Glossopharyngeal (IX cranial) pharyngeal branches.

CONSTRICTOR PHARYNGIS MEDIUS MUSCLE: (MIDDLE CONSTRIC-TOR MUSCLE) A fan-shaped muscle of the pharynx. ORIGIN- From the hyoid bone greater and lesser cornu. DIRECTION- Fanning out backward and medial. INSERTION- On the medial raphe of the pos-terior wall of the pharynx. ACTION- Constricts the pharynx. NERVE- Glossopharyngeal (IX cranial) and Vagus (X cranial) pharyngeal plexus.

CONSTRICTOR PHARYNGIS SUPERIOR MUSCLE: (SUPERIOR CON-STRICTOR MUSCLE) A thin muscle of the pharynx. ORIGIN- Man-dible bone and medial pterygoid plate. DIRECTION- Backward and medial. INSERTION- On the medial raphe of the posterior wall of the pharynx. ACTION- Constricts the pharynx. NERVE-Vagus (X cranial) pharyngeal plexus.

CONTINUANT: Speech sound that retains a relatively steady-state over a period of time.

CONTRACTION PERIOD: The time from the beginning of muscle con-traction to the beginning of muscle relaxation. During this period the muscle performs work.

CONTRALATERAL: On the opposite side.

CONUS ELASTICUS:(CRICOVOCAL MEMBRANE) A band of yellow, elastic tissue connecting the arytenoid, cricoid and thyroid cartilages to each other. It is divided into the anterior ligament, middle cricothyroid ligament, and two lateral or cricothyroid membranes.

CONVEX: A rounded surface like an outer segment of a sphere.

CONVOLUTION: A irregular turn or fold such as a gyrus. 2. A fold on the cerebral hemispheres surface.

COPULA: A connecting or a bridging structure.

COPULA LINGUAE: In embryo development, the median ventral elevation on the tongue. Formed by the union of the second branchial arches forming the tongue root.

CORACOID: Shaped like a beak; hook-like.

CORACOID PROCESS: Hook-like process extending upward and laterally from the scapula bone neck.

CORNICULATE: Shaped like a small horn. 2. Cartilaginous nodules located on the arytenoid cartilages of the larynx.

CORNICULATE CARTILAGE: (CARTILAGE OF SANTORINI) Giovamni D. Santorini, Italian anatomist. A conical shaped cartilage nodule of elastic cartilage on the apex of each arytenoid cartilage. It is the articulation point with the top of the arytenoid cartilage.

CORNU: A horn-shaped projection.

CORNU OF THE HYOID BONE: The greater and lesser horns of the hyoid bone.

CORONAL PLANE: (FRONTAL PLANE) Anatomical plane dividing the body into back and front portions.

CORONAL SUTURE: The junction formed by the frontal and parietal bones.

CORONOID: Crown-shaped.

CORONOID PROCESS: A process on the mandible bone ramus, directed somewhat posterior with the anterior surface convex, the posterior border concave. The lateral surface is the insertion point for the temporalis muscle.

CORPORA QUADRIGEMINA: The inferior and superior cilliculi on the posterior surface of the mesencephalon (midbrain).

CORPUS: The body of a organ or structure. pl. corpora.

CORPUS CALLOSM: A white band of interconnecting nerve fibers joining the two hemispheres of the brain.

CORPUS STRIATUM: Consists of the caudate and lentiform nuclei, and the fibers of the internal capsule between them. Located in the cerebral hemispheres.

CORPUSCLE: A small body or mass, applied to the specialized cell bodies in blood or bone.

CORTEX: Outer layer or an organ or substance. 2. The outer layer of the brain (cerebral cortex) or bone. pl. cortices.

CORTI'S GANGLION: (AUDITORY GANGLION) (SPIRAL GANGLION) The collection of elongated nerve cells which pass from the modiolus to the organ of Corti.

CORTI'S CANAL: (CORTI'S TUNNEL) A triangle-shaped canal, within the organ of Corti. Its shape is formed by the basilar membrane as the base, and the two side are formed by the pillars, or rods, of Corti.

CORTICOBULBAR FIBERS: (CORTICOSPINALIS FIBERS) Fibers which form the spinal cord corticospinal tract.

CORTICOSPINAL SYSTEM: (PYRAMIDAL PATHWAY) (PYRAMIDAL TRACT) Either of the three decending tracts of the spinal cord.

CORTOCOPONTINE FIBERS: Fibers in the cerebral cortex which synapse on the same side of the brain.

COSTAL: Pertaining to the rib. 2. The cartilage that connects the rib to the sternum bone.

COSTAL ANGLE: The point where the lower border of the false ribs and the axis of the sternum bone meet.

COSTAL CARTILAGE: Cartilage which connects a true rib with the sternum bone, or the end of a rib with the costal cartilage above.

COSTAL GROOVE: (COSTAL SULCUS) Located on the inferior and internal portion of a rib bone containing the intercostal nerve and vessels.

COSTAL NOTCH: Located on the lateral surface of the sternum bone for articulation of the costal cartilages. The costal notches consist of seven pair.

COSTAL PLEURA: (PARIETAL PLEURA) Serous membrane lining the walls of the thoracic cavity.

COXA: The hip or hip joint. pl. coxae.

cps: Abbreviation for cycles per second.

CRANIAL: (CEPHALAD) (ROSTRAD) Toward the head or superior portion of the body.

CRANIAL NERVES: The twelve pair of nerves arising from the brain stem and classified as mixed, motor or sensory and named to describe their distribution, function or nature and consist of the following:

I	Olfactory- sensory	VII	Facial- mixed
II	Optic -sensory	VIII	Vestibulocochlear- sensory
III	Oculomotor-motor	IX	Glossopharyngeal- mixed
IV	Trochlear- motor	X	Vagus- mixed
V	Trigeminal-mixed	XI	Accessory- motor
VI	Abducens-motor	XII	Hypoglossal-motor

CRANIAL PART-ACCESSORY NERVE: A motor portion of the accessory (XI cranial) nerve directed to the larynx, levator veli palatine muscle and uvula.

CRANIOSACRAL DIVISION-AUTONOMIC NERVOUS SYSTEM: (PARASYMPATHETIC DIVISION- AUTONOMIC NERVOUS SYSTEM) This division is connected to the central nervous system by efferent fibers from the facial (VII cranial), glossopharyngeal (IX cranial), vagus (X cranial) nerves and fibers from the second, third and fourth sacral segment of the spinal cord and are usually located peripherially near the structures they serve. This system tends to act to restore reserves by slowing the heart beat and the alimentary tract and glands become more active and is the innervator of involuntary muscle, directed to the eye muscles, glands of the gums, lips, salivary glands and soft palate.

CRANIUM: (SKULL) The bony framework of the head consisting of eight cranial bones, housing, and protecting,the brain. One each of the ethmoid, frontal, occipital and sphenoid, and two each of the parietal and temporal. Fourteen facial bones for the framework for most of the speech mechanism consisting of one each of the mandible and vomer and two each of the inferior conchae, lacrimal, maxilla, nasal, palatine and zygomatic bones.

CRESCENDO: The gradual increase in intensity or loudness.

CREST: A prominent ridge.

CRETINISM: A congenital lack of thyroid secretion.

CRIBRIFORM: Perforated with tiny holes like a sieve.

CRIBRIFORM PLATE-ETHMOID BONE: (HORIZONTAL PLATE) A thin perforated partition, of the medial portion of the horizontal plate, of the ethmoid bone between the cranium and nasal cavities. It is held in place by the ethmoidal notch of the frontal bone and roofs the nasal cavities. The plate is narrow and deeply grooved on each side; it supports the olfactory bulb and contains a passage for the olfactory nerves.

CRIBROSA MEDIA: An area in the internal auditory canal with openings for nerves directed to the saccule.

CRIBROSA SUPERIOR: An area in the upper portion of the internal auditory canal containing small foramen for passage of nerves to the semicircular ducts and utricle.

CRICOARYTENOID JOINT: A synovial (diarthrodial) joint which permits lateral and gliding movement of the arytenoid cartilages. Consists of a fibrous articular capsule with a synovial membrane lining.

CRICOARYTENOID LIGAMENT-ANTERIOR: Extends from the anterolateral base of the arytenoid to the cricoid cartilage restricting the backward movement of the arytenoid cartilage.

CRICOARYTENOID LIGAMENT-POSTERIOR: Extends from the base, and muscle process, of the arytenoid cartilage to the cricoid cartilage lamina. Restricts the forward motion of the arytenoid cartilage.

CRICOARYTENOID MUSCLE-LATERAL:(LATERAL CRICOARYTENOID) A broad fan-shaped intrinsic adductor of the larynx. ORIGIN- The upper surface of the cricoid cartilage. DIRECTION- Upward and backward. INSERTION- Arytenoid cartilage muscular process. ACTION- Brings together the vocal folds. NERVE- Vagus (X cranial) laryngeal and recurrent branches.

CRICOARYTENOID MUSCLE- POSTERIOR: (POSTERIOR CRICOARY-TENOID) A broad intrinsic abductor muscle of the larynx. ORIGIN- The posterior portion of the cricoid cartilage. DIRECTION- Upward and lateral. INSERTION- Arytenoid cartilage muscular process. ACTION- Rotation and seperation of the vocal folds. NERVE- Vagus (X cranial) laryngeal and recurrent branches.

CRICOID: Ring or signet shaped.

CRICOID CARTILAGE: The lowermost, signet ring-shaped, hyaline cartilage immediately superior to the first tracheal ring. The broad lamina faces posterior with a vertical ridge at mid-line dividing two shallow depressions. The ridge serves for attachment of the esophagus muscle fibers, and from the shallow depressions originate the posterior cricoarytenoid muscle. On each side of the anterior arch a small facet articulates with the thyroid bone inferior cornu. This permits the cricoid or thyroid to rotate, which is a portion of the pitch changing mechanism. The superior border contains the cricoid notch, located at the midline between two facets, for the bases of the arytenoid cartilages. The cricoid is connected with the first trachea ring by a fibrous membrane, the cricotracheal ligament.

CRICOID LAMINA: A plate extending upward between the posterior border of the thyroid cartilage.

CRICOTHYROID LIGAMENT-MIDDLE: The central portion of the cricothyroid membrane. It is thick, being broad below and narrow above, connecting the front portions of the cricoid and thyroid cartilages. It limits the backward motion of the arytenoid cartilage.

CRICOTHYROID MEMBRANES: (CONUS ELASTICUS) Two membranes from the cricoid cartilage, superior border, extending to the arytenoid cartilages vocal processes and thyroid cartilage angle as free borders.

CRICOTHYROID MUSCLE: A triangular intrinsic muscle of the larynx. ORIGIN- From two muscle groups from the cricoid cartilage anterior and lateral portions as the anterior pars recta and caudal pars oblique. DIRECTION- pars recta vertical upward, pars oblique vertical backward. INSERTION-pars recta, Thyroid cartilage lamina.

Pars oblique thyroid cartilage inferior cornu. ACTION-Lengthen, stretch and tense vocal folds. NERVE- Vagus (X cranial) superior laryngeal branch.

CRICOTRACHEAL LIGAMENT: (CRICOTRACHEAL MEMBRANE) A thin, fibrous ring connecting the lower portion of the cricoid cartilage with the superior portion of the first tracheal ring.

CRICOVOCAL MEMBRANE: (CONUS ELASTICUS) A band of yellow, elastic tissue connecting the arytenoid, cricoid and thyroid cartilages with each other. It is divided into the anterior ligament, middle cricothyroid ligament, and two lateral or cricothyroid membranes.

CRISTA: A crest or projection.

CRISTA AMPULLARIS: A thickened portion of the membrane lining the ampullae of the semicircular canals covered with neuroepithelium and containing auditory cells.

CRISTA BASILARIS: (BASILAR CREST) A prominence projecting inward, and triangular in shape, from the spiral ligament to which is attached the basilar membrane of the organ of Corti.

CRISTA FALCIFORMIS: A shelf formed of bone dividing the internal auditory canal into portions.

CRISTA GALLI: A smooth, thick, triangular process projecting upward from the ethmoid bone cribriform plate. The falx cerebri, a fold of the dura mater of the brain attaches to it.

CRISTA ILIACA: (ILICA CREST) The superior free border of the ilium bone.

CRITICAL DAMPING: Proposes that, if a mass is displaced it will return to its equilibrium position without overshoot or passing through it, with the return slower as the ratio increases.

CROTAPHION: The tip of the sphenoid bone greater wing.

CROWN: The highest point of a organ or structure. 2. The top portion of a tooth, which projects above the gingivae (gum), covered with enamel.

CRUCIFORM: Cross-shaped.

CRUS: Pillar, or shank, that is leg-like in function or appearance.

2. Either leg of the stapes bone. 3. The long process of the incus.

CUBOIDAL CELL: A epithelial cell having both the height and width equal.

CUL-DE-SAC: A sac-like cavity or tube open only at one end.

CULMEN: The summit, or top. 2. The vermis of the cerebellum between the lobulus centralis and primary fissure. pl. culmina.

CULMEN MONTICULI: Highest lobe of the cerebellum.

CUNEIFORM: Wedge-shaped. 2. Cartilages near the arytenoid cartilages of the larynx.

CUNEIFORM CARTILAGE: (CARTILAGE OF WRISBERG)Heinrich A. Wrisberg, German Anatomist. Two elongated, yellow elastic cartilages, one on each side in the aryepiglottic fold, appearing as small whitish elevations in front of the arytenoid cartilages.

CUNEUS: A wedge-shaped area on the occipital lobe medial surface.

CUPID'S BOW: The shape of the upper lip of the mouth.

CUPOLA: The small dome at the apex of the cochlea and spiral canal. pl. cupulae.

CUPOLA CRISTAE AMPULLARIS: A cap, consisting of a gelatinous mass containing carbonate of lime, over the crista of each ampulla at the opening of each semicircular canal.

CUPOLA SPACE: The tympanic attic. The space above the tympanic cavity (middle ear) proper.

CUPULAR CECUM: The superior blind extremity of the cochlea duct.

CUSP: A pointed or rounded eminence on a tooth surface.

CUTANEOUS: Pertaining to skin.

CUTICLE: The epidermis, 2. A superficial membrane. 3. The hardened layer of skin.

CYMBA: Upper portion of the concha of the ear. 2. Boat-shaped.

CYTOLOGY: The study of cell structures.

CYTON: The cell body of a neuron.

CYTOPLASM: The portion of a cell between the membrane and the nucleus. It contains many well organized structures, organelles (tiny organs) and inclusions. The inclusions have not been shown to serve any useful function.

D

DACRYON: The cranial junction point of the frontal, lacimal and maxillary bones.

DAMPING: To cause a decrease in the amplitude vibration of a form of energy, such as electricity or sound waves.

DARWIN'S TUBERCLE: A projection with a blunt point from the upper portion of the helix of the external ear.

DAUGHTER CELL: A cell formed from the division of a mother cell.

dB: Symbol for decibel. One-tenth of a bel. Used to express loga - rithmic ratio of intensity, power or pressure. It is a 10 x $\log_{10}$ of the ratio between the standard sound exerting a pressure of. 0002 dynes per cm^2 on the tympanic membrane (eardrum) and a com- parison sound.

DEAD AIR: Air in the respiratory tract which does not enter into the carbon dioxide-oxygen exchange. It is located in the larynx, mouth, nasal cavities, pharynx and trachea.

DECIBEL: Symbol- dB. One-tenth of a bel. Used to express loga- rithmic ratio of intensity, power or pressure. It is a 10 x $\log_{10}$ of the ratio between the standard sound exerting a pressure of . 0002 dynes per cm^2 on the tympanic membrane (eardrum) and a com- parison sound.

DECIDUOUS TEETH: (MILK TEETH) (TEMPORARY TEETH) The first set of teeth appearing from approximately the fifth through the thir- ieth month which are shed and followed by the permanent teeth. The twenty teeth include two canine, four incisor and four molar in each jaw represented by the dental formula:

Incisor $\frac{2-2}{2-2}$ Canine $\frac{1-1}{1-1}$ Molar $\frac{2-2}{2-2}$

DECUSSATION: The crossing of fibers connecting unlike centers of the central nervous system. 2. Nerve fibers intersecting in the form of an X.

DEEP:(INTERNAL) Away from the outer surface, toward the inner surface.

DEEP TEMPORAL NERVES: Motor branches of the mandibular nerve,
the third and largest division of the trigeminal (V cranial) nerve
which is directed to the temporalis muscle.

DEFERENT: Carry away from the center.

DEFINITIVE MESODERM: (MESODERM) In embryo development, the
middle layer between the ectoderm and entoderm layers of the primary germ layers from which blood, blood vessels, bone, cartilage,
and connective tissue are derived.

DEGLUTITION: To swallow.

DEITER'S TERMINAL FRAME: The ends of the Deiter's cell flattened-
out where they meet the cells of Hensen to frame the outer wall
of Corti's tunnel.

DEMARCATION: To mark or set limits.

DENRIFORM: Tree-shaped or branch like.

DENDRITE: (DENDRON) Branched and tree-shaped protoplasm from a
nerve cell which receive and communicate impulses toward the
cell body forming synaptic connection with with other neurons.

DENSE BONE: (COMPACT BONE) Bone on the exterior portion of a
bone containing fewer microscopic spaces, being dense and hard.

DENSE FIBROUS TISSUE: The intercellular substance is the major
portion of the structure and contain closely packed fibers. The tissue is divided on the basis of the fibers; white and inelastic (white
fibrous tissue) forming ligaments, tendons and resistant membranes; or yellow and elastic (yellow fibrous tissue) found in some
ligaments and walls of blood vessels such as the large arteries.
This type tissue is found in aponeurosis, ligaments and tendons.

DENTAL ALVEOLI: The cavities of either the mandible or maxilla
bones in which the roots of the teeth are embedded.

DENTAL ARCH: The arch-shaped structure formed by the teeth in
their normal position.

DENTAL CANAL: (ALVEOLAR CANAL) The canals in the maxilla bone
for the communication of blood vessels and nerves to the upper
teeth.

DENTAL CANALICULUS: The tiny channels in tooth dentin, from the cement and enamel to the pulp cavity.

DENTAL FORMULA: Expression of teeth arrangement in the form of a fraction. The mandible (lower) the denominator, and the maxilla (upper) teeth the numerator; with C representing the canine, I the incisor, M the molar and PM premolar.

20 Deciduous	I $\frac{2-2}{2-2}$	C $\frac{1-1}{1-1}$	M $\frac{2-2}{2-2}$	
Teeth				
32 Permanent	I $\frac{2-2}{2-2}$	C $\frac{1-1}{1-1}$	PM $\frac{2-2}{2-2}$	M $\frac{3-3}{3-3}$
Teeth				

DENTAL GERM: The tissues which form the complete tooth. Consists of the dental organ, papilla and sac.

DENTAL LAMINA: In embryo development, a band of epithelial along the gum margin from which the enamel organs develope.

DENTAL NERVE BRANCHES: Sensory branches of the inferior alveolar nerve, a branch of the maxillary nerve, the third and largest division of the trigeminal (V cranial) nerve which forms a nerve plexus within the mandible bone and is directed to the molar and premolar teeth.

DENTAL PAPILLA: A mass of connective tissue which is enclosed by the development of the enamel organ.

DENTAL PULP: Soft, sensitive material containing cells, connective tissue, nerves, and vessels.

DENTAL SAC: The layer of mesenchyma which surrounds the dental papilla and enamel organ.

DENTATUS NUCLEUS: Gray lamina in the hemisphere of the cerebellum, located lateral to the emboliform nucleus. Cells from the dentatus extend to fibers which form a major portion of the brachium conjunctivum.

DENTIFORM: Tooth-shaped.

DENTIN: (DENTINUM) (IVORY) The major substabce or tissue of a tooth, surrounding the tooth pulp and covered with enamel on the crown and on the roots by cementum.

DEOXYRIBONUCLEIC ACID: A complex protein in chromosomes and the chemical basis of heredity factors, also the communicator of genetic information. Abbrivation: DNA.

DEPRESSOR ANGULI ORIS MUSCLE: (TRIANGULARIS MUSCLE) A flat triangular muscle of the face. ORIGIN- Mandible bone near the oblique line. DIRECTION- Vertical, upward. INSERTION- Mouth angle. ACTION- Pulls mouth angle down. NERVE- Facial (VII cranial).

DEPRESSOR LABII INFERIOR MUSCLE: (QUADRATUS LABII INFERIOR MUSCLE; A muscle of the face. ORIGIN- Mandible bone lower border. DIRECTION- Lateral. INSERTION- Lower lip skin. ACTION- Depress lip downward. NERVE- Facial (VII cranial).

DEPRESSOR ALAE NASI: (DEPRESSOR SEPTI MUSCLE) A muscle of the nose. ORIGIN- Maxilla bone incisive fossa. DIRECTION- Upward. INSERTION- The ala and septum. ACTION- Constricts the nostrils and depresses ala. NERVE- Facial (VII cranial) buccal branch.

DERMATOME: A skin area with afferent nerve fibers.

DERMIS: Pertaining to the skin.

DEXTRAL: Pertaining to the right side.

DIAPHRAGM: Located between the abdominal and thoracic cavity. Dome-shaped and slightly higher on the right side than on the left, its origin is at the level of the sixth rib anteriorly and the eleventh or twelfth rib posteriorly. It consists of muscle fibers originating from the margins at the outlet of the thorax.

DIAPHRAGM CONTRACTION: A contraction of the diaphragm pulls the central tendon portion downward and forward, which increases the diameter of the thoracic cavity to increase volume and decrease pressure.

DIAPHRAGM MUSCLE: A muscle of inhalation. ORIGIN- Circumference of the lower thorax; Anterior portion from the ensiform process of the sternum. Lateral portion from the bony and cartilage portion of ribs seven through twelve. Posterior portion from the upper lumbar vertebrae. INSERTION- Central tendon. ACTION- Increases thorax cavity by raising ribs and pulling down on the central tendon. NERVE- Phrenic.

DIAPHYSIS: (SHAFT) A portion of a growing bone. pl. diaphyses.

DIARTHRODIAL: (FREELY MOVABLE JOINTS) Most of the joints of the body that have various degrees and direction of movement. The adjacent ends of the bone are covered with hyaline cartilage. The bones are joined by a ligament lined with a synovial membrane that secretes a lubricant, the articular capsule. They are classified by the kind of movement permitted:

DIARTHRODIAL JOINT		DESCRIPTION
Ball and Socket	(Enarthrosis)-	The round end of one bone fits into the cavity of another. Permits all angular and pivot movement
Condyloid		-Permits all angular movement except axial rotation.
Gliding	(Arthrodia)	-Articular surfaces are concave and convex.
Hinge	(Ginglymus)	-Permits movement in only one direction, either backward or forward.
Pivot	(Trochoid)	- Restricts movement to one axis.
Saddle		- Articular surface of each bone is concave in one direction and convex in the other, permitting all movement except rotation.

DIASTEMA: An empty space between two teeth. 2. A cleft or space. pl. diastemata.

DICHOTOMY: To divide into two.

DIENCEPHALON: (BETWEEN BRAIN) The second portion of the brain between the mesencephalon and telencephalon consisting of the epithalamus, hypothalamus, metathalamus and thalamus. Together with the telencephalon it forms the prosencephalon in embryo development.

DIGASTRIC: To have two bellies. 2. Double bellied muscle near the floor of the mouth.

DIGASTRICUS MUSCLE:A extrinsic suprahyoid larynx elevator. A paired muscle of two bellies united by a rounded tendon.
ORIGIN- Anterior belly- Depression on the mandible bone near the lower border near the symphysis.
Posterior belly- Temporal bone mastoid notch.
DIRECTION- Anterior belly- Down and backward.
Posterior belly- Down and forward.

INSERTION- The two bellies meet at the intermediate tendon on the
hyoid bone.
ACTION- Raises hyoid bone, depresses mandible bone.
NERVE- Anterior belly- Trigeminal (V cranial)
Posterior belly- Facial (VII cranial)

DIGASTRIC NERVE BRANCH: A motor branch of the facial (VII cranial) nerve directed to the posterior belly of the digastricus muscle.

DIGITATE: Having finger-like branches that may intertwine.

DILATION: Process of expanding or enlarging.

DIPHASIC CURVE: The two tracings, or phases, produced by an
oscilloscope.

DIPLOID: To have two sets of chromosomes.

DIRECT PYRAMIDAL TRACT: (VENTRAL CORTICOSPINAL TRACT) A
descending motor tract, near the ventral median fissure in the
cranial portion of the spinal cord, which originates in the precentral motor gyrus and is directed to the mid thoracic level.

DISK: A flat, round structure.

DISORDERS-VOCAL QUALITY: Due to abnormal behavior of vocal
fold patterns; considered to be breathiness, harshness, and hoarse-
ness.

DISPLACEMENT: A measurement of vibratory motion, the difference
between the equilibrium of a body and the later position of that body.

DISTAL: Away from the point of attachment. 2. Away from the midline.

DISTENTION: To stretch apart. To stretch out completely.

DISTOCLUSION: In Angle's classification of malocclusion, Class II:
A retruded mandible bone in relation to the maxilla bone.

DISTOVERSION: The position of the anterior teeth, tilting away from
midline; or the posterior teeth, tilted backward.

DIVERTICULUM: A blind process, tube or sac.

DNA: Abbrivation for deoxyribonucleic acid, a complex protein in
chromosomes and the chemical basis of heredity factors, also the
communicator of genetic information.

DOMINANT HEMISPHERE: The cerebral hemisphere which controls, to a stronger degree, the motor activities such as handedness and speech functions.

DORSAL: Toward the backbone. 2. Away from the front.

DORSAL COCHLEAR NUCLEUS: The cochlear nucleus in the posterior portion of the brain stem.

DORSAL HORN: (POSTERIOR COLUMN) (POSTERIOR HORN) The gray matter of the spinal cord which projects longer and thiner than the ventral horn. It contains sensory cells which receive and relay impulses from the fibers of the spinal nerves for receptor and co-ordination functions.

DORSAL INTERMEDIATE SULCUS: (POSTERIOR INTERMEDIUS SULCUS) Located between the dorsal lateral and dorsal median sulci, the seperation between the cuneatus and fasciculus gracilis.

DORSAL LATERAL SULCUS: (POSTERIOR LATERAL SULCUS) A long, slight furrow which subdivides the spinal cord posterior portion.

DORSAL MEDIAN SEPTUM: (POSTERIOR MEDIAL SEPTUM) A thin sheet of tissue which divides the spinal cord posterior portion into halves.

DORSAL MEDIAN SULCUS: (POSTERIOR MEDIAL SULCUS) A shallow groove where neuroglial tissue extends more than half way into the spinal cord dividing the dorsal portion into left and right halves.

DORSAL ROOT: (SENSORY ROOT) Originates in the dorsal ganglia outside the spinal cord with a single fiber directed into two process-es; one extending to the sensory end of a joint, muscle, or tendon with the other extending into the spinal cord to form the dorsal root.

DORSAL SPINOCEREBELLAR TRACT: An ascending sensory tract with its origin at the third lumbar nerve.

DORSUM: The back convex portion of the tongue, divided at midline into two halves by the median sulcus. The sulcus terminalis is directed forward and lateral, on each side of the tongue margin. The dorsum contains three types of papillae; filiform, fungiform and vallate. 2. The rear and superior surface of a structure.

DORSUM SELLAE: A somewhat square plate of bone forming the pos-terior boundary of the sphenoid bone sellae turcica.

DOUBLE CHIN: (BUCCULA) A fold of fatty tissue under the chin.

DRUM MEMBRANE: The tympanic membrane (eardrum) of the middle ear.

DUCT: A narrow channel or passage with a definate wall and excretion or secretion function.

DUCT OF HENSEN: (DUCTUS REUNIEN) (REUNIENS DUCT) A membranous short tube from the cochlea duct to the saccula in the inner ear which allows interchange of endolymph fluid.

DUCTUS ENDOLYMPHATICUS: A duct extending the membranous labyrinth within the vestibular aquduct to communicate with the inner layer of the dura mater in the cranial cavity.

DUCTS REUNIEN: (DUCT OF HENSEN) (REUNIENS DUCT) A membranous short tube from the cochlea duct to the saccula in the inner ear which allows interchange of endolymph fluid.

DUCTS OF RIVINUS: (SMALL SUBLINGUAL DUCTS) The ducts which drain the sublingual gland, posterior portion.

DURA MATER: The lining of the cranium consisting of a fibrous tough outer layer. One of three membranous layers coverning the brain and spinal cord.

DYNE: A unit of energy necessary to accelerate one gram of material one centimeter per second per second.

DYNE PER SQUARE CENTIMETER: (dyne/cm^2)(MICROBAR) A unit for measurement of sound pressure. The amount of energy necessary to accelerate one gram of material one centimeter per second per second.

E

EAR: The organ of balance and hearing which is divided into three portions: External ear- the outer part the pinna, external auditory canal and the outer surface of the tympanic membrane (eardrum. The tympanic cavity (middle ear)- containing the malleus, (hammer), incus (anvil) and stapes (stirrup) bones, the ossicular chain, the inner surface of the tympanic membrane (eardrum) and the auditory (Eustachian) tube. The inner (internal) ear-contains the semicircular canals, cochlea and vestibule.

EAR BONES: The three smallest bone of the body, forming the ossicular chain of the tympanic cavity (middle ear). Consists of the malleus (hammer), incus (anvil) and stapes (stirrup) bones.

EARDRUM: (TYMPANIC MEMBRANE) A membrane which seperates the external auditory canal from the tympanic cavity (middle ear). The eardrum is disk-like, a three layer structure that extends obliquely downward and inward. The layers consist of the outer layer; a continuation of the skin lining the auditory canal; the inner most layer is mucous membrane lining the tympanic cavity; the central layer is fiberous, with fibers arranged both concentrical and radial that provide the resilient, thin connective tissue for strength. The top portion of the eardrum lacks the central layer and is lax, the pars flaccida. The rest of the eardrum has the central layer, being more stiff, the pars tensa.

EAR DUST: (OTOCONIA) (OTOLITHS) Minute dust-like particles of calcium carbonate in one layer in the maculae of the inner ear. As head position changes the particles roll against hair cells to send nerve impulses to the brain as to body orientation and equilibrium.

EAR LOBE: The small lobe on the lower portion of the external ear. It has no known function.

EAR WAX: (CERUMEN) A soft secretion found only in the external auditory canal. It serves as a protective device for self cleansing of the ear.

ECTETHMOID: The lateral mass of the ethmoid bone.

ECTODERM: Outermost layer of the three layers of protoplasm that form a cell membrane. In embryo development this layer forms the nervous systems, skin and special sense organs.

EDDY CURRENT: Current running contrary to the main current. 2. A circular, or contrary current.

EDEMA: Abnormal collection of tissue fluids causing swelling.

EDENTULOUS: The loss of natural teeth. 2. Toothless.

EDGE TONE: Method of setting the air in a column into vibration by blowing a stream of air over a sharp edge.

EFFERENT: To carry away from a center or organ, such as efferent nerves carring impulses from the brain or spinal cord to the periphery.

EFFERENT FIBER: Carrier of outgoing impulses, such as motor nerves.

EFFERENT NERVOUS SYSTEM: (AUTONOMIC NERVOUS SYSTEM)(INVOLUNTARY NERVOUS SYSTEM) A division of the nervous system, an efferent (motor) system with fibers divided into two divisions. The parasympathic (craniosacral)division containing visceral efferent fibers which originate from the medulla and sacral portion of the spinal cord and the sympathetic (thoracolumbar) division receiving visceral fibers from a chain of fibers of the cell ganglia, one on each side of the spinal cord. The parasympathic division is associated with regulation processes and body maintenance and repair during the state of body rest. The sympathic division takes precedence and is dominant in emergency and stress situations by acceleration of heart beat, shutting off body activities such as digestion and diverting the blood supply to the peripheral muscular system for the flight or fight response.

ELASTIC CARTILAGE: Appears yellow, due to a large number of yellow elastic fibers, is flexable, and the ground substance contains collagenous fibers. It is found in the auditory tube, epiglottis and external ear to strengthen and maintain shape.

ELASTIC TISSUE: A form of connective tissue which is composed of a large number of yellow elastic fibers. Found in some ligaments and the walls of large arteries.

ELASTICITY: Property of returning to original form subsequent to removal of a deforming force.

ELECTRODES: The surface of contact between a metallic and a nonmetallic conductor. 2. A terminal through which electrical energy is applied to or away from the body.

ELECTROMYOGRAM: A record of the potential difference between two points on the skin resulting from the activity, or action potential, of a muscle. The action is usually a wave form of the muscle contraction as a result of electrical stimulation from the nervous system.

ELECTROMYOGRAPH: Instrument for measuring and recording electrical potentials generated by active muscles.

ELECTROMYOGRAPHY: The recording and interpretation of muscle tissue electrical activity. Abbreviation; EMG.

ELECTROTONUS: The changed condition of conductivity and excit- ability of a muscle or nerve between the two electrodes when a current is applied to any portion of its length.

ELEIDIN: A material similar to protoplasm in the cells of the stratum lucidum of the vermilion skin.

ELLIPTICAL RECESS: A depression on the medial wall of the vestibule which contains the utricle.

EMBOLIFORM: Wedge-shaped.

EMBOLIFORM NUCLEUS: A small mass located between the dentate nucleus and the globosus nucleus receiving fibers from the vermis and sending fibers into the brachium conjunctivum.

EMBRYO: Development stage in humans from conception through approximately the eighth week.

EMBRYOLOGY: Stude of the development of the embryo.

EMBRYONIC DISK: In embryo development, a flat area in the ovum where the first traces of the embryo are visible.

EMG: Abbreviation for electromyography. The interpretation of muscle tissue electrical activity.

EMINENCE: A projection or prominence, such as on a bone surface.

ENAMEL: The dense, extremely hard, white substance forming a cover which protects the dentin portion of the crown of a tooth.

ENAMEL BUILDER: (AMELOBLAST) Cylinder shaped epithelial cell in the tooth enamel, the inner most layer from which enamel is made.

ENARTHROSIS JOINT: (BALL AND SOCKET JOINT) A type of diarth - rodial joint where the round end of one bone fits into the cavity of another. Permits angular and pivot movements in all directions.

ENDBRAIN: (TELENCEPHALON) In embryo development, the anterior portion of the prosencephalon from which the cerebral hemispheres and corpora striata develop. Along with the diecephalon it forms the prosencephalon.

END BRUSH: (TELODENDRIA) The many, highly-branched, tiny, filament terminations of an axon.

END FOOT: (TERMINAL BUTTON) An enlargement of a fibril at the point of synapse where it makes contact with another cell.

END ORGAN: The structure at the termination of a nerve fiber which changes stimulus into nervous activity, such as the organ of Corti in the cochlea.

ENDOCRINE SYSTEM: A electrochemical system of ductless glands that discharge their secretions (hormones) directly into the blood stream, playing a role in energy and growth. The glands include the adrenals, ovaries or testes, pancreas, parathyroid, thymus and thyroid.

ENDODERM: In embryo development, the innermost layer of cells of the embryo lining the digestive and respiratory tracts.

ENDODELIAL CELL: A flat cell that forms the lining membrane of vessels.

ENDOLYMPH: (SCARP'S FLUID) Antonio Scarpa, Italian Physician. Pale, watery, fluid within the saccule, scala media (cochlea duct), semicircular canals and utricle secreted by the stria vascularis.

ENDOLYMPHATIC DUCT: (ENDOLYMPH DUCT) A canal connecting the endolymphic sac with the membranous labyrinth. It ends in temporal bone petrous portion as a pouch, the endolymphatic sac.

ENDOMYSIUM: A thin sheath of connective tissue, meshlike, which invest each strated muscle fiber and bind them together.

ENDOTHELIAL TISSUE: Composed of one layer of squamous (flat) cells that make a smooth surface coverning the inner lining of the blood and lymph vessels.

ENDONEURIUM: A sheath of connective tissue which seperates individual nerve fibers.

ENDPLATE: A flattened structure where motor nerves terminate at the ending of a motor nerve fiber which is involved in the communication of nerve impulses to the muscles.

ENSIFORM: (XIPHOID) Sword-shaped.

ENSIFORM CARTILAGE: (ENSIFORM PROCESS) XIPHOID CARTILAGE)

The lowest sword-shaped portion of the sternum bone.

ENTODERM CELLS: The inner most layer of the three germ layers of the embryo which form the epithelial lining of the digestive and respiratory tracts, tympanic cavity (middle ear) and auditory tube, and a major portion of the tonsils.

ENTRANCE TO THE TYMPANIC ANTRUM: A large irregular opening leading backward from the epitympanic recess into a large air space, the tympanic antrum which communicates with the mastoid air cells.

ENZYME: A protein which is capable of producing chemical changes in other substances without changing itself.

EPENDYMA: The membranous lining of the central canal of the spinal cord and ventricles of the brain.

EPENDYMAL CELL: Cells lining the ependyma, the lining of the central canal of the spinal cord and ventricles of the brain.

EPENDYMAL LAYER: In embryo development, the inner layer of the neural tube wall bounding the central canal which consists of the floor and roof plates.

EPIDERMIS:The outer, nonvascular, nonsensitive layer of the skin. Consist of five layers from outer to within; stratum corneum; stratum lucidum; stratum granulosum; stratum spinosum and stratum basale.

EPIGLOTTIS: A leaf-shaped, lid-like, structure of yellow elastic cartilage which projects upward behind the tongue root to cover the entrance to the larynx when swallowing. The stem portion is covered by mucous membrane, attached to the thyroid cartilage below the superior notch by the thyroepiglottic ligament. It is attached at the broadest point to the hyoid bone body by a elastic band, the hyoepiglottic ligament. The anterior surface is covered by mucous membrane forming three glossoepiglottic folds. The two lateral folds are partially attached to the pharynx wall, and the medial fold is anterior to the tongue root at midline. The function is, by reflex, to cover the larynx entrance while food passes on the way to the esophagus. It may change laryngeal tone due to changes in the shape and size of the laryngeal cavity.

EPIMYSIUM: The fibrous outer sheath of connective tissue surrounding an entire muscle.

EPINEPHRINE: (ADRENALINE) A hormone produced by the adrenal gland medulla portion. The effect is like those produced by the sympathetic division of the autonomic nervous sustem.

EPIOTIC: Located above, or on the ear.

EPIPHYSIS: End of a long bone, wider than the shaft. Composed of cartilage, or separated from the shaft by a cartilage disk. pl. epi-physes.

EPITHALAMUS: The portion of the thalamencephalon posterior, and superior to the thalamus. It consist of the habenula, habenular commissure, pineal body, and trigonum habenulae.

EPITHELIAN CELL: Cells forming epithelial surfaces of membrane and skin.

EPITHELIAL TISSUE: Composed of closely packed cells arranged in a continuous sheet of one to several layers with shapes either squa-mous, (flat) or columnar (rod-like) with little intercellular sub-stance. It covers surfaces of organs, forms the outer layer of skin, lines canals and cavities, and forms ducts, tubes and portions of secreting glands.

EPITHELIUM: The outer layer of cells forming the epidermis of the skin, covering the internal and external surfaces of the body. The cells are joined by a cementing substance. It is formed into a simple single layer, or stratified several layers. Epithelium is clas-sified into types on the basis of cell shape and number of layers deep.

EPITYMPANIC RECESS: (ATTIC) (RECESSUS EPITYMPANICUS) The superior portion of the tympanic cavity (middle ear) above the ty-panic membrane (eardrum) containing the malleus (hammer) bone head and incus (anvil) bone short limb.

EPONYM: A person from whom a place or structure takes its name.

EQUILIBRIUM: State of balance or rest. 2. The state of air particle at rest with no displacement.

ESOPHAGUS: A muscular canal extending from the pharynx to the stomach. pl. esophagi

ESTOGEN: Hormone produced by the ovaries. Responsible for development of secondary sexual characteristics.

ETHMOID: Sieve-like.

ETHMOID BONE: A complex, light, sieve-like, spongy bone which projects down from between the orbital plates of the frontal bone, and forms a portion of the walls of the nasal and orbital cavities. It consists of four portions, the cribriform plate (horizontal plate), perpendicular plate (vertical plate) and two lateral masses, and the middle and superior nasal conchae. It contains a number of thin walled cavities, the ethmoidal cells which open into the nasal cavity. Articulation is with the frontal, inferior nasal concha, lacrimal, maxilla, palatine, sphenoid and vomer bones.

ETHMODIAL CANAL: Two grooves between the frontal and ethmoid bones across the lateral portion of the ethmoid bone to the cribiform plate.

ETHMOIDAL NERVE: The anterior and posterior sensory branches of the nasociliary nerve, which is a branch of the ophthalmic nerve, the first division of the trigeminal (V cranial) nerve directed to the ethmoidal and frontal sinuses.

ETHMOIDAL NOTCH: Located on the orbital portion of the frontal bone. It separates the two orbital plates and contains and cribiform plates of the ethmoid bone.

ETHMOID SINUSES: (ETHMOID AIR CELLS) Numerous thin walled cavities in the ethmoid bone between the upper portions of the nasal cavities and orbits. They are arranged on each side into three groups anterior, middle, and posterior. The anterior and middle groups open into the middle passage of the nose, the posterior group open into the superior passage. Development is early in fetal life.

EUSTACHIAN TUBE: (AUDITORY TUBE) (TUBA PHARYNGOTYMPANICA) Bartolomno Eustachio, Italian Anatomist. A canal from the tympanic cavity (middle ear) by which it communicates with the nasal portion of the pharynx. It is lined with mucous membrane and formed from bone, cartilage and fibrous tissue divided into the cartilaginous, ishmus, membranous and osseous portions. It provides for equalization of air pressure between the middle ear and outside air without rupture to the tympanic membrane (eardrum) and allows drainage of normal and diseased secretions from the middle ear into the nasopharynx.

EUSTACHIAN CUSHION: (TORUS TUBARIUS) A ridge of cartilage covered with ciliated mucous membrane behind the pharyngeal opening of the Eustachian tube.

EVAGINATION: To grow outward.

EVERSION: A turning outward.

EXCITATION TIME: (CHRONAXIE TIME) Time required for the excitation of a nervous element by a definite stimulus. 2. Minimum time at which current just doubles the rheobase and excite contraction.

EXISE: To remove a part, organ or foreign material.

EXOPHTHALMOS: Abnormal protrusion of the eyeball from the orbit cavity.

EXPIRATION BREATHING: (EXHALATION BREATHING) Expulsion of air from the lungs until the inside and outside pressures are equal.

EXPIRATORY FORCES: Gravity, tissue elasticity, and torque, used in quiet breathing.

EXPIRATORY RESERVE VOLUME: (RESERVE AIR) (SUPPLEMENTAL AIR) The amount of air that can be forcible exhaled after a normal exhalation.

EXTENSION: Movement that brings members of a limb toward a straight condition as, the angle between the two bones is increased.

EXTENSOR: Muscles responsible for producing extension.

EXTERNAL: (SUPERFICIAL) Toward the surface. 2. Farther from the midline.

EXTERNAL AUDITORY CANAL: The canal leading from the external ear to the tympanic membrane (eardrum) which allows sound waves to reach the middle and inner ear.

EXTERNAL AUDITORY CANAL NERVE BRANCHES: Sensory branches of the auriculotemporal nerve, a branch of the mandibular nerve, the third and largest division of the trigeminal (V cranial) nerve. Directed to the skin lining of the external auditory canal and tympanic membrane (eardrum).

EXTERNAL AUDITORY CANAL CARTILAGE: The cartilage that forms

the wall for a portion of the canal.

EXTERNAL CAPSULE: A layer of white matter which forms the corpus striatum border.

EXTERNAL HAIR CELLS: Hair cells along the organ of Corti of the inner ear. In three rows, they are longer than the inner hair cells and serve as recepters for sound stimulus.

EXTERNAL INTERCOSTAL MUSCLES: Muscles of the thorax and of inhalation. ORIGIN- From the outer portion of the lower border of each rib. DIRECTION- Front- Obliquely downward and forward. Back- Downward and outward in back. INSERTION- Upper border of each rib below. ACTION- Draw ribs together and raise. NERVE- The intercostals, consisting of thoracic nerves one through eleven.

EXTERNAL LARYNGEAL NERVE BRANCH: A motor branch of the superior laryngeal nerve, a branch of the vagus (X cranial) nerve, directed to the cricothyroid muscle and a portion of the inferior pharyngeal constrictor muscle.

EXTERNAL MEDULLARY LAMINA: A layer of gray matter under the stratum zonale, a white layer of the thalamus. It is divided into anterior, lateral, and medial portions.

EXTERNAL NASAL NERVE BRANCHES: Sensory branches of the infraorbital nerve, a branch of the maxillary nerve, the second division of the trigeminal (V cranial) nerve directed to the skin of the nose.

EXTERNAL OBLIQUE MUSCLE:A abdominal muscle of exhalation. ORIGIN- From the exterior surface and lower borders of ribs number five or six through twelve. DIRECTION- Downward and medial. INSERTION- Abdominal aponeurosis, and iliac crest. NERVE- The intercostals, consisting of thoracic nerves five through twelve.

EXTERNAL OCCIPITAL PROTUBERANCE: A protuberance at the junction of the head and neck, near midline of the occipital bone squama.

EXTERNAL PTERYGOID MUSCLE: (PTERYGOIDEUS LATERALIS) A thick cone-shaped muscle of Mastication. ORIGIN- From two heads; the lower or inferior from the pterygoid plate lateral surface and the upper or superior from the sphenoid bone Great wing. DIRECTION- Backward and horizontal. INSERTION- Mandible bone condyle. ACTION- Moves mandible bone side to side, opens jaw, protudes jaw. NERVE- Trigeminal (V cranial) mandible branch.

EXTERNAL THYROARYTENOID MUSCLE: (THYROMUSCULARIS MUSCLE) A portion of the thyroarytenoid muscle located parallel to the vocalis muscle, inserting into the thyroid lamina.

EXTEROCEPTIVE: The external field of distribution of receptor organs.

EXTEROCEPTOR: A sensory end organ for the reception of outside stimuli.

EXTRAEMBRYONIC MESODERM: In embryo development, the middle germ layer of the blastocryst cavity. Located outside of the embryo it is a portion of the fetal accessory organs.

EXTRAPOLATE: To estimate a quantity by extending the given data farther than the established known range.

EXTREMITY: A limb of the body.

EXTRINSIC: Originating outside a organ, part or structure.

EXTRUDE: To push; to extend outward.

EXUDATE: A discharge of fluid tissue.

EYE TEETH: (CANINE TEETH) The four teeth, one on either side of each jaw, between the incisors and molars with a cone-shaped crown and a single root; used for tearing. Approximate eruption: Deciduous 18-24 months, Premanent 12-14 years.

F

f: Abbreviation for frequency. The number of double vibrations or cycles per second (cps) or hertz (Hz) of a sound wave.

FACE: The anterior portion of the head from the chin to the forehead, inclusive.

FACET: A plane surface on a structure.

FACIAL ANGLE: The point where the nasal spine and external auditory canal meet, between the upper middle incisor teeth.

FACIAL BONES: Bones forming the facial portion of the skull consisting of the hyoid, mandible, maxilla, palatine, and zygomatic bones.

FACIAL CANAL: (AQUEDUCT OF FALLOPII) A canal through which the facial (VII cranial) nerve passes, located in the temporal bone petrous portion. It is directed between the cochlea and semicircular canals, directed above the fenestra vestibuii (oval window) then down along the area of mastoid cells to the stylomastoid foramen, continuing to divide into two branches at the posterior border of the mandible bone ramus.

FACIAL MUSCLES ANGULAR: Consists of the depressor labii inferior (quadratus labii inferior), levator labii superior (quadratus labii superior), and zygomaticus muscles.

FACIAL MUSCLES PARALLEL: Consists of the incisivis labii inferior, incisives labii superior, and platysma muscles.

FACIAL MUSCLES VERTICAL: Consists of the canine (levator anguli oris), mentalis (levator menti), and triangularis (depressor anguli oris) muscles.

FACIAL NERVE: (FACIALIS NERVE) VII cranial, a mixed nerve with the motor fibers from a nucleus in the lower portion of the pons. The sensory fibers from a geniculate ganglion on the facial nerve. The distribution is into central and peripheral fibers. The central fibers pass into the medulla oblongata and end in the terminal nucleus of the glossopharyngeal (IX cranial) nerve. The peripheral fibers form the sensory root and emerge from the brain with the motor root. Behind the mandible bone ramus the facial nerve divides into many branches to serve most of the muscles of facial expression; the auricle, buccinator, platysma, stapedius, styohyoid, scalp and the posterior belly of the digastric muscle. The sensory areas served are; taste in the anterior two thirds of the tongue and the soft palate.

FACIAL NUCLEUS: A group of cells in the pons from which the facial (VII cranial) nerve arises.

FALCIFORM: Sickle-shaped.

FALLOPIAN AQUEDUCT: (FALLOPIAN CANAL) A bony canal containing the facial (VII cranial) nerve. It crosses the wall of the tympanic cavity (middle ear) above and behind the fenestra vestibuli (oval window) and curves downward along the mastoid wall.

FALSE GLOTTIS: (RIMA VESTIBULI) The space between the left and right vestibular folds of the larynx above the true vocal folds.

FALSE RIBS: (VERTEBROCHONDRAL RIBS) The five lower ribs on each side not directly attached to the sternum bone.

FALSE VOCAL FOLDS: (VENTRICULAR FOLDS) Two folds of thick mucous membrane above the vocal folds (true vocal folds). Each fold encloses a thin band of fibrous tissue, the ventricular ligament. The folds move with the arytenoid cartilages and are farther apart than the true vocal folds. They usually do not function in normal voice production but function in holding of the breath, providing moisture for the true vocal folds and protecting the larynx when swallowing.

FALX CEREBRI: A small fold of dura mater extending downward into the longitudinal fissure between the cerebral hemispheres.

FASCIA TISSUE: A dense fibrous membrane coverning, seperating and supporting muscles arranged in sheets or sheaths. pl. fasciae.

FASCICULUS: A bundle of muscle or nerve fibers. pl. fasciculi.

FASCICULUS CUNEATUS: The ascending tract of the spinal cord seperated from the fasciculus gracilis tract by the dorsal intermediate septum. It arises from the posterior toots and terminates in the nucleus gracilis of the medulla, carrying sensations of joint, muscle and tendon movements and tactile and vibration sensations, (proprioceptive sensation).

FASCICULUS GRACILIS: The ascending tract of the spinal cord located next to the dorsal median septum running through the entire cord. It arises from the posterior roots and terminates in the nucleus gracilis of the medulla, carrying sensations of joint, muscle and tendon movement, and tactile and vibration sensations, (proprioceptive sensation).

FASTIGIAL NUCLEUS: A mass of gray matter located over the roof of the fourth ventricle in the cerebellum medial to the globase nucleus. It receives fibers trom the vestibular branch of the auditory (VIII cranial) nerve and directs efferent fibers into the brain stem.

FASTIGIUM: In the shape and being pointed. 2. Coming to a point.

FAT: A white or yellow adipose tissue which forms between organs of the body.

FAUCES: (ISTHMUS FAUCIUM) A narrow passage from the mouth to the pharynx. Bounded superiorly by the soft palate, posteriorly the dongue dorsum, and on each side by the glossopalatine arch.

FAUCIAL ISTHMUS: The opening into the pharynx.

FENESTRA: A small opening, or a small window in a bony structure, usually closed by a membrane. 2. The oval and round windows of the tympanic cavity (middle ear). pl. fenestra e.

FENESTRA ROTUNDA: (ROUND WINDOW) A round opening into the base turn of the cochlea located in the tympanic cavity (middle ear) medial wall (labyrinthic wall). The opening is closed by a thin membrane, the secondary tympanic membrane.

FENESTRA VESTIBULI: (OVAL WINDOW) A kidney-shaped opening in the tympanic cavity (middle ear) medial wall (labyrinthic wall). It is located above the fenestra rotunda (round window) and opens into the vestibule of the inner ear.

FIBER: A thin strand, or nerve or muscle tissue.

FIBRIL: A thread-like component of a fiber.

FIBRIL MUSCLE: A very minute fibril in the cytoplasm of smooth muscle cells.

FIBRIL NERVE: Delicate fibrilis in a cell body. 2. An axon.

FIBROBLAST: A long flat, cell with processes at each end. A cell from which connective tissue developes.

FIBROUS ASTROCYTE: An adult neuroglia cell with small, long and smooth branch like expansions.

FIBROUS CARTILAGE: Composed of collagenic fibers. It is found in joints and portions of the sponal column.

FIBROUS MEMBRANE: (PERIOSTEUM) The covering of bones, except at articulating surfaces. The external layer contains numerous blood vessels and the internal layer larger connective tissue cells. It serves as a support structure for blood vessels and attachment of ligaments, muscles and tendons.

FIBROUS TISSUE: Connective tissue consisting of fibers. There are three types; areolar, white fibrous and yellow fibrous.

FILIFORM: Thread-shaped.

FILIFORM PAPILLA: The minute size filiform-shaped papellae on the anterior two thirds of the tongue.

FILUM: A thread-like structure.

FILUM TERMINALE: A thin, thread-like band which extends through the vertebral canal from the conus medullaris down to the coccyx, to which it attaches.

FIRING: The movement of a nervous impulse by a receptor.

FIRST ORDER NEURONS: Nerve fibers directed from the cochlea to the dorsal and ventral cochlear nuclei in the auditory pathway.

FISSION: Cleaving; splitting into parts.

FISSURE: A deep furrow, groove, or natural division in the cerebral hemispheres of the brain. 2. A division or a lung. 3. A break in the enamel of a tooth. pl. fissurae.

FISSURE OF GLOTTIS: (RIMA GLOTTIDIS) An enlongated fissure between the true vocal folds in front, and the bases and vocal ligaments of the arytenoid cartilages behind. Its shape and width depend on the arytenoid cartilages and true vocal folds during phonation and respiration. The anterior membranous portion, approximately three fifths the length, is the membranous (vocal) glottis bounded laterally by the muscular portion of the vocal folds. It extends from the anterior commissure of the true vocal folds to the vocal process of the arytenoid cartilages. The cartilaginous glottis is the posterior portion and is bounded by the vocal processes and medial surfaces of the arytenoid cartilages. The length, width, and shape, of the glottis differs from person to person.

FISSIRE OF ROLANDO: (CENTRAL SULCUS) Divides the frontal and parietal lobes of each cerebral hemisphere. It begins at approxi-mately midline between the inferior and superior borders and directed up and backward to its termination near the midline of the superior border.

FISSURE OF SYLVIS: (LATERAL FISSURE) Francois Sylvius, French Anatomist. A fissure which seperates the temporal lobe from the frontal and parietal lobes of the brain. It begins at the inferior border and courses backward and up to terminate on the lateral surface.

FISTULA: Abdnormal communication or passage between internal organs, or from an internal organ to the outside. Sometimes made for the purpose of taking body fluids for lab study. pl. fistulae.

FIXATION: Holding in a immobile position. 2. To fasten, hold, or suture, in place.

FIXATION MUSCLES: Muscles which act to maintain the body in a specific position.

FIXATION THEORY: Proposes that the tympanic musculature supplements the suspending ligament in maintaining the correct position of the occicles of the tympanic cavity (middle ear). The ossicular chain consisting of the malleus (hammer), incus (anvil), and stapes (stirrup) bones, move back and forth to transfer sound impulses to the fenestra vestibuli (oval window), and prevents the chain from passing specific critical limits of movement.

FLACCID: Soft, weak. 2. Muscles that have lost their quality or tone.

FLEXION: Bending or being bent. The angle between two bones is decreased with flexion.

FLEXOR: Muscle that will flex at a joint.

FLOATING: To move about, not firmly attached.

FLOTING RIBS: (VERTEBRAL RIBS) The two pair of lower ribs, numbers eleven and twelve, not attached to the sternum bone by costal cartilage.

FLOCCULENT: Containing downy or flaky masses.

FLOCCULONDULAR LOBE; Consists of the flocculi and vermis modulus.

FLOCCULUS: A small lobe below and behind the center oeduncle of the cerebrum on each side of the median fissure. pl. flocculi.

FLOOR PLATE: (VENTRAL PLATE) In embryo development, the longitudinal zone forming the neural tube floor.

FLUX: A discharge or flow that is in excess.

FOLIUM: A leaflike structure. pl. folia.

FOLLICLE: A gland or sac which is capable of secretion.

FOOTPLATE: The base of the stapes (stirrup) bone that rest in the fenestra vestibuli (oval window).

FORAMEN: A opening or passage in a bone that is a natural part of the bone. pl. foramina.

FORAMEN CECUM: A depression near the tongue root, at midline.

FORAMEN LACERUM: An opening at the base of the medial pterygoid plate. The inferior portion being filled with fibrocartilage formed by the junction of the occipital bone basilar portion, sphenoid bone great wing, and the temporal bone petrous portion.

FORAMEN MAGNUM: (OCCIPITAL MAGNUM) The large oval opening in the occipital bone connecting the cranial cavity with the vertebral canal. It is used for the passage of the accessory nerves, medulla oblongata, and vertebral arteries.

FORAMEN OF MONRO: (INTERVENTRICULAR FORAMEN) Alexander Monro, Scottish Anatomist. An opening between the lateral and third ventricle.

FORAMEN OBTURATOR: The large opening between the pubis and ischium bones.

FORAMEN OVALE: An opening in the sphenoid bone great wing posterior margin, for passage of the mandibular division of the trigeminal (V cranial) nerve.

FORAMEN ROTUNDUM: A round opening on the medial surface of each great wing of the sphenoid bone, for passage of the maxillary branch of the trigeminal (V cranial) nerve.

FORAMEN SPINOUS: The opening in the sphenoid bone great wing for passage of the meningeal artery.

FORAMEN VENA CAVA: Opening in the diaphragm, at the junction of the middle and right leaflets, at the level of the eighth thoracic vertebra through which the inferior vena cava and phrenic nerve pass.

FORAMINA OF SCARPA: Two openings in the maxilla bone palatine process, at midline, for passage of the nasopalatine nerve.

FORCE: The physical action capable of moving, or modifying, body motion. 2. Energy or power which starts or stops motion.

FORCES OF EXHALATION: Forces acting on exhalation, including elasticity of tissue, gravity, and torque.

FOREBRAIN: (PROSENCEPHALON) The anterior portion of the brain, developed from the three divisions of the embryo neural tube. It consists of the posterior dienecphalon (between brain) portion consisting of epithalamus, hypothalamus, metathalamus, thalamus, subthalamus, and anterior portion of the telencephalon (endbrain), consisting of the cerebral cortex composed of the cerebral hemispheres and lamina terminalis, the corpus striatum and rhinencephalon.

FOREGUT: In embryo development, the organ from which the esophagus, pharynx, and stomach develop.

FOREHEAD: The portion of the head between the eyes and hairline, formed by the anterior portion of the frontal bone.

FORMANT: Special partial tone of constant pitch for each vowel.

FORNIX: A space or structure shaped like a arch or vault.

FORNIX BODY: The area under the corpus callosum, formed by the middle portion of the fornix.

FOSSA: A hollow or pit.

FOSSA INCUDIS: A small depression in the lower and back portion of the tympanic attic which holds the incus (anvil) bone short process.

FOSSA OF ROSENMULLER: (PHARYNGEAL RECESS) Johann C. Rosemuller, German Physician. A deep depression in the pharynx wall above and behind the auditory (Eustachian) tube.

FOURTH ORDER NEURONS: Nerve fibers directed from the inferior colliculus to the medial geniculate body in the auditory pathway.

FOURTH VENTRICLE: A flat, diamond-shaped cavity containing spinal fluid and communicating with the third ventricle by the aqueduct of Sylvius. It is bounded by the cerebellum behind, and the medulla oblongata and pons in front, it is the remains of the cavity of the embryo neural tube.

79

FOVEA: Depression or pit-shaped. pl. foveae.

FRENULUM: Small fold of mucous membrane that checks or limits the movement of a part. pl. frena.

FREQUENCY: Abbreviation f; The number of double vibrations or cycles per second (cps) or hertz (Hz) of a sound wave.

FREQUENCY THEORY: (TELEPHONE THEORY) William Rutherford. Proposes that the basilar membrane of the cochlea vibrates as a complete unit like the telephone diaphragm. The analysis of pitch perception occuring not in the cochlea but in the auditory (VIII cranial) nerve with the frequency of the impulse directed in each nerve fiber to the auditory area, the transverse temporal gyrus, of the brain.

FRICATIVES: Continuant sounds that have a friction-like quality, caused by the release of sound through a narrow opening between the organs of articulation. The breath is maintained with pressure to make the sounds continuous.

FRONT: The functional portion of the tongue below the hard palate.

FRONTAL: A anatomical plane, side to side, dividing into front and back parts.

FRONTAL BONE: A single bone consisting of the horizontal, or orbital portion, and the vertical squama portion, composed of two thin plates, forming the vaults of the orbits, which are seperated by the ethmoidal notch into which the ethmoid bone cribriform plate fits. It contains the frontal sinus and serves as the insertion point for major muscles of speech.

FRONTAL EMINENCE: A rounded elevation located on the frontal bone squama portion on either side of the metopic suture.

FRONTAL INFERIOR GYRUS: Located on the frontal lobe, external surface, of the cerebrum between the inferior frontal sulcus and sylvian fissure.

FRONTAL LOBE-CEREBRUM: The anterior portion of the cerebral cortex in front of the central sulcus and on the convex side. Consists of four convolutions, the inferior, frontal, middle frontal, superior frontal and precentral.

FRONTAL MIDDLE GYRUS: On the frontal lobe between the inferior and superior frontal sulcus.

FRONTAL NERVE: A sensory nerve. The largest of the three branches of the ophthamic nerve, the first division of the trigeminal (V cranial) nerve. It divides into the supraorbital branch directed to the forehead, and the supratrochlear branch directed to the lower portion of the forehead.

FRONTAL NOTCH: Located on the frontal bone, for transmission of the supraorbital nerve.

FRONTAL PLANE: (CORONAL PLANE) Anatomical plane dividing the body into back and front portions.

FRONTAL PROCESS-MAXILLA BONE: A strong bony plate directed upward, medial and posteriorly. Forms the lateral frame of the nose, and the medial surface contributung to the nasal cavity lateral wall.

FRONTAL PROCESS-ZYGOMATIC BONE: (FRONTAL SPHENOIDALIS PROCESS-ZYGOMATIC BONE) The thick process which articulates with the frontal bone zygomatic process, and the sphenoid bone great wing.

FRONTAL SINUS: Irregular air cavity in the frontal bone, on each side, behind the superciliary arch. They are seperated by the midline bony septum, and communicate with the middle passage of the bony nasal cavity on the same side. They reach their full size after puberty.

FRONTAL SPINE: A sharp, pointed porcess directed downward from the nasal process of the frontal bone.

FRONTAL SUPERIOR GYRUS: Located on the frontal lobe, above the superior frontal sulcus.

FRONTAL SUTURE: The line between the left and right halves of the frontal bone.

FRONTOMAXILLARY SUTURE: The line between the frontal bone and maxilla bone frontal process.

FRONTO-NASAL DUCT: A passage into the frontal sinus which opens into the anterior portion of the passage.

FRONTONASAL PROCESS: In embryo development, the expansion of the facial process into the bridge of the nose and forehead.

FRONTOSPHENOIDAL PROCESS-ZYGOMATIC BONE: The process is

thick and tooth-like, articulating with the frontal bone zygomatic process.

FUNCTIONAL RESERVE VOLUME: Functional air in the lungs that can be expelled.

FUNDAMENTAL FREQUENCY: The major component of a wave, with the reference point being either the greater amplitude or lowest frequency. The ratio between fundamental frequency and vocal fold vibration is I:I.

FUNDIFORM: Loop or sling shaped.

FUNDUS TYMPANIC: (JUGULAR WALL) A thin plate of bone that forms the floor of the tympanic cavity (middle ear). It separates the cavity from the groove containing the jugular vein.

FUNGIFORM: Fungus or mushroom shaped.

FUNGIFORM PAPILLA: Large, rounded-shaped papilla found on the apex and sides of the tongue.

FUNICULUS: A portion or structure resembling a cord. 2. Cord-like.

FURCULA: In embryo development, an elevation in the floor of the pharynx which develops into the aryepiglottic folds and epiglottis.

FURROW: A groove.

FUSIFORM: Spindle-shaped.

FUSIFORM CELL: A spindle-shaped cell.

FUSION: The process of joining together.

G

GAMETE: One of two cells, male or female, whose union is necessary, in sexual reproduction, to begin the growth of a new human.

GAMETOGENESIS: Development of male and female sex cells.

GANGLION OF SCARPA: (VESTIBULAR GANGLION) Antonio Scarpa, Italian Anatomist. The sensory ganglion of bipolar cells of the vestibular division of the auditory (VIII cranial) nerve with its fibers arising from the cristae of the ampullae of the semicircular ducts, saccule, and utricle.

GANGLION RIDGE: (NEURAL CREST) In embryo development, a cellular band lateral to the neural tube for the origin of the spinal
ganglia and sympathic division of the autonomic nervous system.

GASTRIC: Pertaining to the stomach.

GENIAL: Pertaining to the chin.

GENICULATE: A sharp bend. 2. Bent like a knee.

GENICULATE GANGLION: A small mass forming the sensory ganglion of the facial (VII cranial) nerve where the nerve changes
direction. It divides further into branches of the greater petrosal
nerve directed to the soft palate.

GENICULUM: A knee-like bend in a small organ or structure. pl.
genicula.

GENIOGLOSSUS MUSCLE: A large flat extrinsic muscle of the tongue.
ORIGIN- Mandible bone mental spine. DIRECTION- Fan-like.
INSERTION- Hyoid bone, dorsum of the tongue. ACTION- Depress
and protrude tongue. NERVE- Hypoglossal (XII cranial).

GENIOHYOID MUSCLE: A extrinsic suprahyoid larynx elevator. A
barrow muscle above the medial border of the mylohyoid muscle.
ORIGIN- Mandible bone mental spine. DIRECTION- Backward and
downward. INSERTION- Hyoid bone body. ACTION- Pulls hyoid bone
up and forward. NERVE- Hypoglossal (XII cranial).

GENU: Point of joining between the leg and thigh (femur). pl. genua.

GIANT PYRAMIDAL CELLS: (BETZ CELLS)Viadimir A. Betz, Russian
Anatomist. Large pyramidal ganglion cells forming layer V of the
cerebral cortex six cell layer.

GIGANTISM: The abnormal overgrowth of the body, or a part of
the body.

GILL CLEFTS: (BRANCHIAL GROOVES) In embryo development, a
number of slight furrows which seperate the branchial arches.

GINGIVAE: (GUM) The mucous membrane tissue which covers the
crown of unerupted teeth, and surrounding the neck of erupted
teeth. pl. gingiva.

GINGLYMUS JOINT: (HINGE JOINT) Type of diarthrodial joint which
permits movement in one direction, either backward or forward.

GIRDLE: A confining, or encircling structure.

GLABELLA: The smooth portion of the frontal bone above the nose, lying between the superciliary arches.

GLADIOLUS: Body or main portion. 2. The body or major portion of the sternum bone.

GLAND: A cell, tissue, or organ which produces and secretes a substance used elsewhere in the body.

GLENOID: Shaped like a pit or socket.

GLENOID FOSSA: (MANDIBULAR FOSSA) A depression in the surface of the temporal bone squama portion, at the base of the zygomatic process, in which the mandible bone condyloid process rest.

GLENOID FOSSA- SCAPULA: A depression on the scapula for articulation with the humerus bone.

GLIA: A glue-like tissue or structure. 2. The supporting tissue of the brain and spinal cord.

GLIDING JOINT: (ARTHRODIA JOINT) A type of diarthrodial joint where the articular surfaces are alternately concave and convex.

GLOBOSE: Globe, or spherical shaped.

GLOBOSUS NUCLEUS: A mass of gray matter in the cerebellum, located between the nucleus emboliform and nucleus fastigal, which receives fibers from the vermis and sends efferent fibers to to the red nucleus.

GLOBULAR PROCESSES OF HIS: In embryo development, the development of the face, nose, and rounded lateral angles of the medial process.

GLOBUS PALLIDUS: A small medial, pale portion of the lentiform nucleus. It is separated from the putmen by the external medullary lamina, and is divided into the external and internal portions by the medial medullary lamina.

GLOSSOEPIGLOTTIC FOLDS: Three folds of mucous membrane extending from the epiglottis to the tongue base.

GLOSSOPALATINE ARCH: (ANTERIOR PILLAR OF FAUCES) (PALATO-GLOSSAL ARCH) The anterior of the two folds of mucous membrane formed by the downward curve from the soft palate to the side of the tongue base, enclosing the palatoglossal muscle.

GLOSSOPALATINE MUSCLE: (PALATOGLOSSUS MUSCLE) A muscle of the soft palate. ORIGIN- Soft palate anterior surface. DIREC — TION- Downward, forward and lateral, INSERTION- Side of the tongue. ACTION- Raises tongue, constricts the fauces. NERVE- Vagus (X cranial) pharyngeal plexus.

GLOSSOPALATINE NERVE: (NERVUS INTERMEDIUS) A portion of the facial (VII cranial) nerve, between the facial nerve root and the auditory (VIII cranial) nerve, containing both parasympathetic and sensory fibers.

GLOSSOPHARYNGEAL NERVE: (GLOSSOPHARYNGEUS NERVE) A motor and sensory nerve distributed to the pharynx and tongue with the origin between the inferior cerebellar peduncles and olive. Directed laterally it exits the cranium through the jugular foramen. At the location of the jugular foramen two enlargements, the inferior and superior ganglia of the nerve divide into the carotid, pharyngeal, and tympanic major branches. The origin of the carotid branch is just after the nerve exits from the jugular foramen down the carotid artery to the carotid sinus. The pharyngeal branch con- sist of three or four fibers which join the vagus (X cranial) nerve and are directed to the pharynx muscles and mucous membrane. The tympanic origin of the nerve is from the inferior portion of temporal bone petrous portion, directed through and opening near the medial wall of the tympanic cavity (middle ear) to the tensor tympanic muscle by the semicanal. It supplies the mucous mem- brane of the tympanic cavity with sensory fibers.

GLOTTAL: A consonant classification of articulators used, and the position they are in. Sound is made by the breath coming through the opening between the true vocal folds and without modification by other articulators.

GLOTTAL ATTACK: (GLOTTAL STROKE) The release of the adductor muscles to suddenly initiate vocal fold vibration.

GLOTTAL CHINK: (FISSURE OF GLOTTIS) (RIMA GLOTTIDIS) An enlongated fissure between the true vocal folds in front, and the bases and vocal ligaments of the arytenoid cartilages behind. Its shape and width depend on the arytenoid cartilages and true vocal folds during phonation and respiration. The anterior membranous portion, approximately three fifths the length, is the membranous (vocal) glottis bounded laterally by the muscular portion of the vocal folds to the vocal process of the arytenoid cartilages. The cartilaginous glottis is the posterior portion and is bounded by the vocal processes and medial surfaces of the arytenoid cartilages. The length, width, and shape, of the glottis differs from person to person.

GLOTTAL STOP: The sudden stopping of vocal fold vibration by contraction of the adductor muscles to suddenly release air with an explosive effect.

GLOTTIS: The true vocal folds and the elongated fissure between them, the rima glottis. The glottis is the apparatus of the larynx for sound production. A leaf-shaped, lid-like fibrocartilage, the epiglottis, protects the opening.

GLOTTIS SPURIOUS: The false glottis. The ventricular folds.

GLUCAGON: A secretion of the pancreas gland which speeds the breakdown of glycogen and the release of glucous by the liver.

GLUTEUS MAXIMUS: The large muscle of the buttock. Its origin is on the lateral surface of the ilium.

GOBLET CELL: A epithelial cell containing mucus which bulges out.

GOITER: An enlargement of the thyroid gland.

GOLGI APPARATUS: Camillo Golgi, Italian Histologist. Irregular structures in nerve cells which change during Wallerian degeneration.

GOLGI CELLS: Nerve cells in the cerebral cortex and the posterior horns of the spinal cord. Classified as Type I, that have long axons which pass out of the gray matter and Type II, having short axons which do not pass out of the gray matter.

GOLGI COMPLEX: Located in secretory cells on the secretion side of the cell. It functions in the preparation and storage of secretory material.

GOMPHOSIS: A type of synarthrosis joint where a conical process fits into a socket in an immovable joint.

GONADS: The sex glands. Ovaries in the female and testes in the male.

GRAAFIAN FOLLICLE: Regnier de Graff, Dutch Anatomist. A follicle beginning at puberty in the female which develops monthly. Each one contains an ovum which is released from the ovary.

GRANULAR LAYER: The cell layer of the cerebral cortex containing small nerve cells (granule cells), and Goli Type II cells.

GRAY COMMISSURE: The strip which connects the dorsal and lateral columns of the spinal cord into a H shape.

GRAY FIBERS: (NAKED FIBERS) (REMAK FIBERS) Robert Remak, German Neurologist. Unmyelinated nerve fibers in the gray matter of the brain and spinal cord with the majority found in the autonomic nervous system.

GRAY MATTER: Nervous tissue containing large amounts of neuron cell bodies. Includes portions of basal ganglia, cerebral cortex, H-shaped area around the spinal cord, nerves, and sympathetic ganglion.

GRAY RAMI FIBERS: Communicating branch of nerve bundles of the sympathetic ganglia and communicated by spinal nerves to arteries, and veins.

GREAT WING- SPENOID BONE: Two large processes of bone which are lateral and upward from the sides of the spenoid bone body. The inferior surface forms a large portion of the orbital wall with the superior surface forming a portion of the medial cranial fossa.

GREATER ALAR: Two flexible cartilages of the nose forming the lateral and medial walls.

GREATER CORNU: The large horns of the hyoid bone.

GREATER PALATINE NERVE: A sensory branch of the pterygopalatine nerve which is a branch of the maxillary nerve, the second division of the trigeminal (V cranial) nerve directed to the ethmoidal and sphenoidal sinuses.

GREATER PETROSAL NERVE: (GREATER SUPERFICIAL PETROSAL NERVE: A sensory branch of the facial (VII cranial) nerve directed to the soft palate.

GREATER PALATINE FORAMEN: (MAJOR PALATINE FORAMEN: The opening at either posterior angle of the hard palate for passage of the palatine nerve.

GREATER SCIATIC NOTCH: A large notch on the os coxae (hip bone) posterior border containing the sciatic foramen through which the sciatic nerve passes.

GROOVE: A shallow depression or furrow.

GROUP A FIBERS: (ALPHA NERVE FIBERS) The largest of the anterior horn motor cells of the somatic nervous system with a conduction speed of appooximately one hundred meters per second.

GROUP B FIBERS: (BETA NERVE FIBERS) Fibers of the autonomic nervous system with a conduction speed of approximately 4. 5 meters per second.

GROUP C FIBERS: (GAMMA NERVE FIBERS) Fibers of the somatic nervous system with a conduction speed of approximately twenty meters per second.

GUM: (GINGIVAE) The mucous membrane tissue which covers the crown of unerupted teeth and surrounds the neck of erupted teeth. pl. gingiva.

GUTTUR: The throat.

GYRUS: One of many convolutions, or gyri, of the cerebral hemispheres of the brain. They are separated by deep grooves (fissures) or shallow grooves (sulci).

H

HABENULA: A narrow bandlike structure. pl. habenulae.

HABITUAL PITCH: (NATURAL LEVEL) (PITCH LEVEL) The laryngeal tone that varies in pitch over a music range of two octaves. This level is located approximately one-fourth up the total singing range.

HAIR: A very thin thread-like filament.

HAIR CELL: A specific sensory cell, with one end having cilia (hairlike projections) which are in contact with or imbedded in the tectorial membrane of the organ of Corti. The other end is in contact with numerous nerve endings. 2. Specific sensory cells within the semicircular canals and vestibule of the inner ear serving the balance organs.

HALITUS: The expired breath.

HAMMER: (MALLEUS BONE) The first and largest ossicle attached to the tympanic membrane (eardrum), and to the incus (anvil) bone by a diarthrodial joint. It consist of the head, neck, the anterior, lateral and manubrium processes.

HAMULUS: A hook shaped process. 2. The process which forms a portion of the boundry of the helicotrema, a small opening at the apex of the cochlea through which the scala tympani and scala vestibuli communicate. 3. A process on the sphenoid bone medial pterygoid plate inferior portion. The tendon of the tensor veli palatine muscle is directed around the process.

HAPLOID: To have a single set of chromosomes.

HARD PALATE: (PALATUM DURUM) The anterior rigid portion of the palate formed by the medial projection of the maxilla bone palatine processes. Meeting at midline it forms approximately three quarters of the bony roof of the mouth, which forms the floor of the nasal cavity. It is covered by mucous membrane and rugae (small ridges or wrinkles).

HARMONIC THEORY: Charles Wheatstond, British Physicist. Proposes that the reed tone is complex with many harmonics of the fundamental frequency. The vouel heard results from the augmentation of specific harmonic components of the reed tone.

HARMONICS: Composed of the fundamental frequency and overtones when the frequencies are multiplers of the fundamental frequency.

HARSHNESS: A vocal quality disorder usually caused by irregular vocal fold vibration due to excessive tension of the vocal folds. Phonation is initated by glottal attack.

HAVERSIAN CANAL: Clopton Havers, British Physician. One of several minute channels in compact bone which carry nutrients.

HEAD: In bone, an enlargement at one end of the body, beyond the neck. 2. The portion of the body containing the brain and sense organs.

HEAD OF MALLEUS: (MALLEI CAPITULUM) The superior portion of the malleus bone containing the facet for articulation by a diarthrodial joint with the incus (anvil) bone.

HELICIS MAJOR MUSCLE: An intrinsic large muscle of the external ear. ORIGIN- Spine of the helix. INSERTION- Anterior rim of the helix. ACTION- Tenses skin of the auditory canal. NERVE- Facial (VII cranial) temporal branch, posterior auricular branch.

HELICIS MINOR MUSCLE: An intrinsic small muscle of the external ear. ORIGIN- Anterior rim of the helix. INSERTION- Concha. NERVE- Facial (VII cranial) temporal and posterior auricular branches.

HELICOTREMA: The opening at the apex of the cochlea through which the scala tympani and scala vestibuli communicate. The opening allows for the displacement of perilymph fluid to the fenestra vestibuli (round window) as a sound stimulus is received.

HELIX: Rim-like margin of the external ear. 2. A coil or spiral.

HEMISPHERE: Either the left or right half of the cerebellum.

HENSEN'S BODY: Victor Hensen, German Anatomist. A modification of a Golgi net in the organ of Corti hair cells.

HENSEN' S CELLS: Tall supporting cells on the outside of the Deiters cells. Positioned in four to six rows, with small bases expanding toward their apex, which forms the outer most coverning of the organ of Corti.

HENSEN'S NODE: (PRIMITIVE NODE) In embryo development, a group of cells at the cephalic end of the primary groove from which the notochord developes.

HENSEN'S STRIPE: Dark band on the under surface of the tectorial membrane of the organ of Corti.

HERTZ: Heinrich Hertz, German Physicist. A unit of frequency equal to one cycle per second. Abbreviation: Hz.

HESCHL'S GYRUS: (TRANSVERSE TEMPORAL GYRUS) Richard L. Heschl, Austrian Physician. The auditory reception center (area 41-42) below the Sylvis fissure of the temporal lobe.

Hg: Chemical symbol for mercury, a metallic element in a liquid state at ordinary temperatures.

HIATUS: A cleft, gap, or opening.

HIATUS ESOPHAGEUS: Oval-shaped opening, posterior to the middle portion of the central tendon, on the diaghragm surrounded by contracting muscle fibers through which the esogphagus and vagus (X cranial) nerve pass.

HILLOCK AXON: A cone shaped expansion at the point where the axon attaches to a nerve cell body.

HILTON MUSCLE: (ARYEPIGLOTTICIS MUSCLE) John Hilton, English Surgeon. Muscle fibers located next to the laryngeal saccule. Its origin is the arytenoid apex, becoming less defined and inserting on the epiglottis lateral surface, Its action compresses the saccule whose secretion lubricates the surface of the true vocal folds.

HILUS: Depression or pit where nerves and vessels enter. pl. hili.

HINDBRAIN: (RHOMBENCEPHALON) In embryo development, the hindbrain which divides into the metencephalon and myelencephalon. Including the cerebellum, medulla oblongata, and pons.

HINGE JOINT: (GINGLYMUS) A type of diarthrodial joint which permits movement in one direction, either backward or forward.

HIP: The articulation point of the femur and innominate bones on either side of the pelvis.

HIP BONES: INNOMINATUM) (OS COXAE) Consists of three major portions; ilium, ischium and pubis. pl. ilia, ischia, pubes.

HIPPOCAMPUS: A curved structure in the floor of the inferior horn of the lateral ventricle.

HIPPOCAMPAL FISSURE: A fissure extending from the posterior portion of the corpus callosum to the temporal lobe tip.

HISTOLOGY: The stude of tissues.

HOARSNESS: A vocal quality disorder usually caused by laryngitis, the swelling and thickening of the vocal folds causing irregular vibration of the vocal folds and incomplete glottal closure.

HOOKE'S LAW: Robert Hooke. Proposes within limits of perfect elasticity distortion in elastic solids is proportional to the distorting force, The amount a spring balance is stretched is directly in propositioned to the amount of force applied.

HORIZONTAL: (TRANSVERSE) Anatomical plane, across, dividing

into upper and lower parts.

HORIZONTAL CELLS OF CAJAL: Santiago R. Cajal, Spanish Histologist. A neuroglia cell in the molecular layer of the cerebral cortex.

HORIZONTAL PART: (ORBITAL) The portion of the frontal bone composed of the two orbital plates which are seperated by the ethmoid notch that receives the ethmoid bone cribriform plate. The plates form the vaults of the orbital cavity.

HORIZONTAL PLATE: (CRIBRIFORM PLATE- ETHMOID BONE) A thin perforated partition, of the medial portion of the horizontal plate, of the ethmoid bone between the cranium and nasal cavities. It is held in place by the ethmoidal notch of the frontal bone and roofs the nasal cavities. The plate is narrow and deeply grooved on each side; It supports the olfactory bulb and contains a passage for the olfactory nerves.

HORIZONTAL PLATE- PALATINE BONE: The quadrilateral shaped portion of the palatine bone. Its inferior concave surface forms a portion of the hard palate and the concave superior surface forms a portion of the nasal cavity floor.

HORMONE: Chemical secreation of the endocrine gland. Carried by body fluid, it regulates the function of another gland.

HUMERUS: Bone in the upper arm from the elbow to the shoulder.

HUSCHKE'S AUDITORY TEETH: (AUDITORY TEETH) Emil Huschke, German Anatomist. Tiny toothlike projections on the vestibular, or inner edge, of the organ of Corti.

HUSSON'S THEORY: Raoul Husson. Proposes that each vibratory cycle of the vocal folds is initated by a nerve impulse transmitted from the brain to the vocalis muscle by the vagus (X cranial) nerve recurrent branch.

HYALIN: The major substance of hyaline cartilage, being a translucent substance.

HYALINE CARTILAGE: Composed of collagenous fibers that form a fine network and appear as a blue-white glass-like substance. With are it turns yellow and cloudy and calcification may occur. Flexible, and slightly elastic, it is found in the costal cartilages, septum of the nose, and forms the framwork for the bronchi, larynx and trachea. The cartilage surface is covered by a membrane of fibrous connective tissue (perichondrium).

HYDRATE: Containing water.

HYDRAULIC THEORY: Proposes that the movement of the stapes bone inward produces positive pressure in the cochlea causing the basilar membrane to bulge. The bulge travels from base to apex to accept the displacement of fluid caused by the stapes. As the stapes bone moves negatively outward the second displacement begins at the base traveling to the apex. Senstation of pitch depending upon the spread of the displacement on the different length of the basilar membrane.

HYOEPIGLOTTIC LIGAMENT: A extrinsic, elastic, triangular shaped band with the base attached to the superior border of the hyoid bone body and the tip connected to the anterior superior surface of the epiglottis.

HYOGLOSSAL MEMBRANE: A fibrous plate connecting the hyoid bone to the under surface of the tongue.

HYOGLOSSUS MUSCLE: An extrinsic muscle of the tongue. ORIGIN-Hyoid bone greater cornu. DIRECTION- Vertical upward. INSER-TION- Side of the tongue. ACTION- Depress tongue. NERVE-Hypoglossal (XII cranial).

HYOID ARCH: The second branchial arch in embryo development, from it the hyoid bone lesser cornu, styloid process and stylohyoid ligament form.

HYOID BONE: A somewhat horseshoe-shaped bone in the neck, at the base of the tongue on the level of the third cervical vertebra lying in a horizontal position. It is the point of attachment for the laryngeal muscles, and inferior attachment for the majority of the tongue muscles. Approximately thirty muscles have either their origins or insertion point at the hyoid bone. The majority of the bone consist of the body with the anterior surface convex and the posterior surface concave. On the anterior surface a midline ver-tical ridge divides it into the left and right halves and a tranverse ridge crosses the upper half. On each side of the body a limb, the greater cornu (horn) is directed posteriorly. At the junction of the body and greater cornu a cone-shaped prominence, the lesser cornu is located in line with the transverse ridge of the body.

HYOID CORNU: The greater and lesser horns of the hyoid bone.

HYOID SLING MUSCLES: Muscles which are attached to the hyoid bone, suspending it in position. They include the digastricus (anterior and posterior), geniohyoid, omohyoid, stylohyoid, sternohyoid, sternothyroid, and thyrohyoid.

HYOTHROID LIGAMENT: An extrinsic elastic band from the hyoid bone greater cornu to the superior thyroid cornu.

HYOTHYROID MEMBRANE: A broad fibroelastic sheet arising from the superior border of the thyroid cartilage having fibers directed upward to insert on the posterior surface of the hyoid bone body and greater cornu (horns). The middle portion is thicker and is the middle hyothyroid ligament. The thinner portion contains the internal branch of the superior laryngeal nerve.

HYOTHYROID MUSCLE: (THYROHYOID MUSCLE) A extrinsic infrahyoid muscle of the larynx. ORIGIN- Thyroid cartilage, oblique line. DIRECTION- Vertical, upward. INSERTION- Hyoid bone greater cornu. ACTION- Depress hyoid bone or raise larynx. NERVE- Hypoglossal (XII cranial).

HYPERKINESIA: Excessive movement. 2. Increase which is excessive in motor function or activity.

HYPERTROPHY, The overgrowth or enlargement of an organ or tissue.

HYPOGLOTTIS: The undersurface of the tongue.

HYPOGLOSSAL CANAL: A canal in the occipital bone lateral portion for the passage of the hypoglossal (XII cranial) nerve.

HYPOGLOSSAL NERVE: (HYPOGLOSSUS) XII cranial, a motor nerve of efferent fibers for the muscles of the tongue. The deep origin is from the hypoglossal nucleus and the superficial origin is from the medulla onlongata. Exit is through the hypoglossal canal, directed downward between the internal carotid artery and jugular vein , branching out to the first cervical nerve.

HYPOPHARYNX: The lowest portion of the pharynx which opens into the esophagus and larynx.

HYPOPHYSIS: A process or outgrowth, of the nervous system.

94

HYPOPHYSIS CEREBRI: (PITUITARY GLAND) A ductless gland of the endocrine system located in the sella turcica of the sphenoid bone body. It consists of the anterior and posterior lobes. The anterior lobe secretes six hormones, four of which control activities of the endocrine glands and two controlling growth and metabolism. The posterior lobe contains many nerve pathways from the hypothalamus, the major life regulating center. A hormone (antidiuretic (ADH) secreted by the posterior lobe is responsible for maintenance of the water balance in the body.

HYPOTHALAMUS: A portion of the diencephalon which forms the floor, and a portion of the lateral wall of the third ventricle. It consists of the infundibulm. hypophysis, optic chiasm, and tuber cinereum. Located under the thalamus, it functions in the regulation over water balance and sleep.

I

ILIAC CREST: The superior free margin of the ilium forming the os coxae (hip bone).

ILIAC TUBEROSITY: A rough area on the anterior superior area iliac spine of the ilium bone for the attachment of ligaments and muscles.

ILIOLUMBAR LIGAMENT: A band from the lip of the iliac crest to the transverse processes of lumbar vertebra four and five.

ILIUM BONE: One of the largest bones of each half of the pelvis, the superior and widest part. pl. ilia.

IMMOVABLE JOINTS: (SYNARTHRODIAL JOINTS) Formed by fibrous tissue consisting of four types of joints; gomphosis, schindylesis, suture, and synchondrosis.

IMPEDANCE: The resistance of a electrical or mechanical system to absorption of energy.

IMPEDANCE MATCHING: A connection across a source impedance of another impedance, having the same magnitude and phase.

IMPRESSION: A depression or indentation.

IMPULSE: Activity flowing along nerve fibers.

INCIDENT: Falling upon, with sound or light from the source. Not reflected.

INCIDENT WAVE: A sound wave which strikes a gap in the medium, or strikes a medium which has different reflecting characteristics.

INCISIVE BONE: (INTERMAXILLARY BONE) (PREMAXILLA) A bone forming the median anterior portion of the superior maxilla bone by a thin suture, consisting of the floor of the anterior nasal spine and nose and contains sockets for the incisor teeth.

INCISIVE BRANCH. A terminal branch of the mandibular nerve, the third and largest division of the trigeminal (V cranial) nerve directed to the canine and incisor teeth.

INCISIVE CANAL: A canal in the maxilla bone, from the incisive fossa in the mouth roof to the nasal cavity for transmission of the nasopalatine nerve.

INCISIVE FORAMEN: An opening containing the incisive canal through which the nasopalatine nerve and the descending septal artery pass.

INCISIVE FOSSA: A depression on the anterior surface of the maxilla bone, above the incisor teeth.

INCISIVIS LABII INFERIOR MUSCLE: A small thin muscle of the mouth. ORIGIN- Mandible bone. DIRECTION- Parallel. INSERTION- Mouth angle. ACTION- Draws mouth medial and upward. NERVE- Facial (VII cranial) buccal branches

INCISIVIS LABII SUPERIOR MUSCLE: A flat muscle of the mouth. ORIGIN- Maxilla bone, alveolar border. DIRECTION- Parallel. INSERTION- Mouth angle. ACTION- Draws mouth medial and upward. NERVE: Facial (VII cranial) buccal branches.

INCISIVE NERVE BRANCH: A sensory branch of the inferior alveolar nerve, a branch of the maxillary nerve; the third and largest division of the trigeminal (V cranial) nerve. This forms a nerve plexus within the mandible bone and directed to the canine and incisor teeth.

INCISOR: One of the four front teeth in each jaw, each with a crown shaped like a wedge; used for cutting with a cone-shaped root. Approximate eruption: Deciduous 5-15 months, permanent 7-8 years.

INCUDIFORM: Anvil-shaped.

INCUS BODY: Slightly cubucal, the inside surface contains a deep facet which articulates with the malleus (hammer) bone head.

INCUS BONE: (ANVIL) The middle of the three bones of the tympanic cavity (middle ear) which articulates with the malleus (hammer) bone by a diarthrodial joint. It consist of the body and two processes.

INERTIA: The tendency of a body to remain in a state of rest or of even motion in a straight line.

INFERIOR: (CAUDAL) Below, underneath; toward the hind part of the body.

INFERIOR ALVEOLAR NERVE: A motor and sensory branch of the mandibular nerve, the third and largest division of the trigeminal (V cranial) nerve. It is directed in the mandibke bone to the mental foramen where it divides into the dental, incisive, mental, and mylohyoid branches.

INFERIOR CEREBELLAR PEDUNCLES: (RESTIFORM BODY) Afferent fibers connecting the cerebellum and medulla oblongata and forming the fourth ventricle lateral wall.

INFERIOR COLLICULUS: A bundle of sensory fibers which are directed to the transverse temporal gyrus (area 41-42) the auditory center.

INFERIOR CONSTRICTOR MUSCLE: (CONSTRICTOR PHARYNGIS INFERIOR) A strong, thick muscle of the pharynx. ORIGIN- From the sides of the cricoid and thyroid cartilage. DIRECTION- Backward and medial. INSERTION- On the medial raphe of the posterior wall of the pharynx. ACTION- Constricts the pharynx. NERVE-Vagus (X cranial), pharyngeal plexus.

INFERIOR CORNU: (INFERIOR HORN OF THYROID CARTILAGE) A bony projection directed backward and upward articulating with the cricoid cartilage.

INFERIOR FRONTAL GYRUS: The convolution on the frontal lobe below the inferior frontal sulcus, divided into the anterior, opercular, and triangular portions. The left portion is highly convoluted and referred to as the speech center, Broca's area 44.

INFERIOR GANGLION: (NODOSE GANGLION) An enlargement of the vagus (X cranial) nerve near the jugular foramen. Here the motor and sensory fibers connect with the first and second cervical nerves, hypoglossal (XII cranial) nerve and the sympathetic ganglion.

INFERIOR HORN OF THYROID CARTILAGE: (INFERIOR CORNU) A bony projection, directed backward and upward, articulating with the cricoid cartilage.

INFERIOR NASAL CONCHA: (INFERIOR TURBINATE BONE) A plate of spongy bone scroll-like, forming the inferior portion of the lateral nasal wall. The inferior border forms the lateral and upper boundaries of the inferior nasal canal. It articulates with the ethmoid, lacrimal, maxilla, and palatine bones.

INFERIOR LONGITUDINALIS MUSCLE: A bundle of narrow fibers forming an intrinsic muscle of the tongue between the genioglossus and hyoglosses muscles. ORIGIN- Posterior portion of the tongue, at the base. INSERTION- The tongue tip. ACTION- Pulls the tip down and shortens tongue. NERVE- Hypoglossal (XII cranial).

INFERIOR NUCHAE LINE: The low nuchal line on the outer surface of the occipital bone.

INFERIOR OCCIPITAL GYRUS: The convolutions of the inferior and lateral portion of the occipital lobe on the convex surface.

INFERIOR PALPEBRAL NERVE BRANCHES: Sensory branches of the infraorbital nerve, a branch of the maxillary nerve, the second division of the trigeminal (V cranial) nerve. It is directed toward the skin of the lower eyelid.

INFERIOR TEMPORAL GYRUS: The convolution on the temporal lobe between the inferior temporal and occipitotemporal sulci.

INFERIOR TURBINATE BONE: (INFERIOR NASAL CONCHA) A plate of scroll-like spongy bone forming the inferior most portion of the lateral nasal wall. The inferior border forms the lateral and upper boundaries of the inferior nasal canal. It articulates with the ethmoid, lacrimal, maxilla, and palatine bones.

INFRACOSTAL: Below the ribs, or below a single rib.

INFRAHYOID MUSCLES: Two pair of extrinsic strap-like muscles which support the hyoid bone from below the omohyoid and sternohyoid muscle. The sternothyroid muscle supports from below and is a laryngeal depressor while the thyrohyoid muscle supports from above and is a laryngeal levator.

INFRAORBITAL CANAL: A canal in the maxilla bone, on the floor of the orbit for transmission of the infraorbital artery and nerve.

INFAORBITAL FORAMEN: The opening at the end of the infaorbital canal on the maxilla anterior surface. It transmitts the infaorbital blood vessels and nerves.

INFRAORBITAL GROOVE: The opening in the maxillary bone on the orbital surface for passage of the infraorbital nerve and vessels.

INFRAORBITAL MARGIN- ZYGOMATIC BONE: The inferior entrance to the orbit formed by the infraorbital margin of the maxilla and zygomatic bones.

INFRAORBITAL NERVE: A sensory branch of the maxillary nerve, the second division of the trigeminal (V cranial) nerve. It further divides into the external nasal branch directed to the skin on the side of the nose; inferior palpebral branches directed to the skin of the lower elelid; superior labial branches directed to the labial glands and the skin of the upper lip.

INFRAORBITALIS SUTURE: (TRANSVERSE SUTURE) A fibrous joint directed from the infraorbital foramen to the infraorbital groove.

INFRATEMPORAL FOSSA: (ZYGOMATIC FOSSA) An irregular shaped cavity, medial to the zygomatic arch.

INFRATEMPORAL SURFACE- MAXILLA BONE: Positioned backward and lateral, it is convex and is seperated from the anterior surface by the zygomatic process. The alveolar canals pass through the center and at the lower portion the maxillary tuberosity, a rounded elevation, is prominent after the appearance of the third molar (wisdom tooth).

INFRATROCHLEAR NERVE: A sensory branch of the nasociliary nerve, a branch of the ophthalmic nerve, the first division of the trigeminal (V cranial) nerve, directed to the eyelid and skin on the side of the nose.

INFRAVERSION: Inefficient eruption of a tooth. Failure to reach the gingiva (gum) line.

INFUNDIBULUM: A funnel-shaped hollow mass projecting down-ward and forward to the posterior lobe of the hypophysis cerebri. Forms a portion of the hypothalamus. 2. A funnel-shaped passage.

INGUINAL LIGAMENT: (POUPART'S LIGAMENT) Francois Poupart, French Anatomist. A thin, fibrous band of aponeurosis which joins superiorly with the lower portion of the pectoralis major muscle and sternum bone ensiform process, and inferiorly to the anterior iliac spine and the pubic symphysis.

INHALATION BREATHING: (INSPIRATION BREATHING) Drawing air into the lungs until the insid and outside pressures are equal.

INNER AND OUTER RODS: (PILLARS OF CORTI) Two rows of rod-like bodies, with the inner rods resting on the basilar membrane at an approximate sixty degree angle. The heads of the inner rods contain a hollow which holds the convex portion of the heads of the outer rods. The outer rods, rest on the outer edge of the basilar membrane at an approximate forty degree angle. The heads of the outer rods are shaped like a flat plate containing the phalangeal processes. The phalangeal processes, along with the phalangeal processes of the cells of Deiter, form the delicate net-like reticular membrane.

INNER EAR: (INTERNAL EAR) Consists of the cochlea, semicircular canals, and the vestibule.

INNER HAIR CELLS: The hair cells along the medial side of the inner rods of the organ of Corti.

INNERVATION: The supply to any organ or structure with nerve fibers.

INSCRIPTION: A mark or line.

INSERTION: To implant. 2. Place of attachment of a muscle to the structure that it moves.

INSPIRATION BREATHING: (INHALATION BREATHING) Drawing air into the lungs until the inside and outside pressures are equal.

INSPIRATORY RESERVE VOLUMN: (COMPLEMENTAL AIR: The quant-ity of air which can be inhaled beyond that inhaled during quiet breathing.

INSULA: (CENTRAL LOBE) (ISLAND OF REIL) A triangular shaped area in the cerebral cortex forming the floor of the lateral cerebral fossa.

pl. insulae.

INSULAR: Pertaining to an island.

INSULIN: A secretion of the cells of the Island of Langerhans (the pancreas) essential for maintenance of proper blood sugar level.

INTEGUMENT: Skin. 2. The outer most layer of the body.

INTENSITY: The relative amplitude or strength of electrical, magnetic, or vibrational energy.

INTENSITY CONTROL or PROTECTIVE THEORY: Proposes that muscles contract in a response to specific critical levels of sound intensity. The contraction stops excessive stapes (stirrup) bone vibration by damping the degree of the ossicular chain movement.

INTERARTICULAR: Located between two articulating surfaces.

INTERARYTENOID MUSCLE: (ARYTENOID MUSCLE) An intrinsic adductor on the posterior surface of the arytenoid cartilages. ORIGIN AND INSERTION- Posterior surface and lateral border of one arytenoid cartilage, and inserting into the same area of the opposite cartilage. A complex muscle designated as two portions, the arytenoid oblique and arytenoid transverse.

INTERCOSTAL: Located between the ribs.

INTERCOSTAL NERVES: The first eleven of the twelve thoracic nerves with seperate courses to supply the abdomen and thorax. The twelveth nerve is the subcostal.

INTERDIGITATE: Interlocking or interrelative.

INTERMAXILLARY BONE: (PREMAXILLA) (INCISIVE BONE) A bone forming the median anterior portion of the superior maxilla bone by a thin suture. Consists of the floor of the anterior nasal spine and nose, and contains sockets for the incisor teeth.

INTERMAXILLARY SUTURE: The junction formed between the maxillae bones.

INTERNAL: (DEEP) Away from the outer surface, toward the inner surface.

INTERNAL CAPSULE: A wide band of white matter which seperates the lentiform nucleus from the caudate nucleus and the thalamus. It is shaped at a right angle with the apex, or genu medially directed. The anterior limb is directed lateral and caudal, and contains three types of fibers; corticothalamic fibers from the frontal lobe to the thalamus; frontopontine fibers from the frontal lobe to nuclei of the pons; thalamocortical fibers from the lateral nucleus of the thalamus to the frontal lobe and collaterals from these tracts to the basal ganglia. The genu contains corticobulbar, corticothalamic, and thalamocortical fibers.

INTERNAL EAR: (INNER EAR) Consist of the cochlea, semicircular canals, and vestibule.

INTERNAL GRANULAR LAYER: The fourth layer of the cerebral cortex containing small pyramidal cells and stellate cells.

INTERNAL HAIR CELLS: Hair cells which are in the outer edge of the basilar membrane, the edge nearest the modiolus in the organ of Corti.

INTERNAL INTERCOSTAL MUSCLES: Muscles of the thorax and of inhalation. ORIGIN- Inner portion of the lower border of each rib. DIRECTION- Front- downward and outward, Back-down and inward. INSERTION- Inner portion or the rib below. ACTION- Draw ribs together and raise. NERVE- The intercostals, consisting of thoracic nerves one through eleven.

INTERNAL LARYNGEAL NERVE BRANCH: A sensory branch of the superior laryngeal nerve, a branch of the vagus (X cranial) nerve. It is directed to the aryepiglottic fold, epiglottis and a portion of the tongue base.

INTERNAL LATERAL LIGAMENT: (SPHENOMANDIBULAR LIGAMENT) A thin flat band attached to the inner surface of the mandible bone ramus and the spina angularis of the sphenoid bone.

INTERNAL MEDULLARY LAMINA: A white layer which divides the gray material of the thalamus into the anterior, lateral, and medial portions.

INTERNAL OBLIQUE MUSCLE; An abdominal muscle of exhalation. ORIGIN- Anterior portion of the iliac crest and Poupart's ligament. DIRECTION- Upward and medial. INSERTION- Abdominal aponeurosis, linea albam and ribs eight through twelve. ACTION- Flexes the vertebral column. NERVE- The intercostals, consisting of thoracic nine through twelve.

INTERNAL PTERYGOID MUSCLE: (PTERYGOIDEUS MUSCLE) A thick muscle of mastication. ORIGIN- Lateral pterygoid plate and tuberosity of the maxilla bone. DIRECTION- Downward, lateral and backward. INSERTION- Mandible bone ramus medial surface and angle. ACTION- Closes the jaw. NERVE- Trigeminal (V cranial) mandibular division.

INTERNUNCIAL: A medium of communication between nerve centers and neurons.

INTERNUNCIAL NEURON: (ASSOCIATION NEURON) A central neuron being both afferent and efferent in mediating impulses between a motor and sensory neuron.

INTEROCEPTOR: A receptor activated by internal body stimuli directed to joints, muscles, or tendons.

INTEROSSEUS: A muscle located between bones.

INTERPHASE: In embryo development, the time period when a cell is not dividing. 2. Time between production of a cell and its division.

INTERSTITIAL: In, or between the spaces of tissue.

INTERTRAGAL INCISURE: The small notch between the tragus and antitragus in the external ear.

INTERVAL SCALE: Theoretical basis of a numerical system where the intervals between values are equal, or linear.

INTERVENTRICULAR FORAMEN: (FORAMEN OF MONRO) Alexander Monro, Scottish Anatomist. An opening between the lateral and third ventricle.

INTERVERTEBRAL: Space between the certebrae.

INTERVERTEBRAL DISK: Layers of fibrocartilage substance between bodies of vertebra forming a amphiarthrodial, or yielding joint.

INTERVERTEBRAL FORAMINA: Openings formed by the inferior and superior notches on the pedicles of the vertebra for passage of the spinal nerves and vessels.

INTRA AURAL MUSCLES: The stapedius and tensor tympani muscles in the tympanic cavity (middle ear).

INTRAPULMONARY: In the lungs.

INTRAPULMONIC PRESSURE; Air pressure present within the lungs.

INTRATHORACIC PRESSURE: The air pressure within the thorax.

INTRATHORACIC SPACE: The space between the inner thoracic wall and the lungs. The nonexistance intrapleural space.

INTRINSIC: Located within any given part.

INTRINSIC MUSCLE: A muscle having both its origin and insertion in the same structure.

INVERSION: To turn inward.

INVERTEBRATE: Without a spinal column.

INVESTED: Covered by an outer sheath of connective tissue.

INVOLUNTARY MUSCLE: (CARDIAC) (PLAIN) (SMOOTH) (UNSTRIATED) Muscle which is not under conscious control. Consisting of spin-dly-shpaed cells arranged parallel and grouped into bundles, layers or sheets without the cross striations of other kinds of muscle. It is found in blood vessels and respiratory passages.

INVOLUNTARY NERVOUS SYSTEM: (AUTONOMIC NERVOUS SYSTEM) EFFERENT NERVOUS SYSTEM) A division of the nervous system, an efferent (motor) system with fibers divided into two divisions. The parasympathic (craniosacral) division containing visceral efferent fibers which originate from the medulla and sacral portion of the spinal cord and the sympathetic (thoracolumbar) division receiving visceral fibers from a chain of fibers of the cell ganglia, one on each side of the spinal cord. The parasympathic division is associated with regulation processes and body maintenance and repair during the state of body rest. The sympathic division takes precedence and is dominant in emergency and stress situations by acceleration of heart beat, shutting off body activities such as digestion and diverting the blood supply to the peripheral muscular system for the fight or flight response.

ION: An atom or group of atoms which due to outside force, has lost or gained one or more orbital electrons and has thus become capable of conducting electricity.

IPSILATERAL: On the same side.

ISCHIUM: The lateral, lower portion of the acetabulum, a triangular shaped strong column of bone which decends and ends as a large ischial tuberosity. The inferior portion of the hip bone. pl. ischia.

ISLAND: A cluster of cells.

ISLAND OF LANGERHANS: Paul Langerhas, German Pathologist. A group of irregular cells in the pancrease which produce, and secrete insulin.

ISLAND OF REIL: (CENTRAL LOBE) (INSULA) A triangular shaped area in the cerebral cortex forming the floor of the lateral cerebral fossa.

ISOCORTEX: (NEOPALLIUM) The portion of the cerebral cortex which is non-olfactory, composed of six layers of cell and fiber tissue.

ISOTONIA: The same activity, tension or tone. 2. A muscle contraction where equal tension is maintained while the muscle length is decreased.

ISTHMUS: A narrow passage between two cavities.

ISTHMUS PORTION- AUDITORY TUBE: The narrowest portion of the auditory tube.

ISTHMUS FAUCIUM: (FAUCES) A narrow passage from the mouth to the pharynx. Bounded superiorly by the soft palate, posteriorly by the dorsum of the tongue, and on each side by the glossopalatine arch.

ITER CHORDAE ANTERIUS: (CANAL OF HUGUIER) Pierre C. Huguier, French Surgeon. A canal through which the chorda tympani nerve exits the tympanic cavity (middle ear).

IVORY: (DENTIN) (DENTINUM) The principle substance or tissue of a tooth, surrounding the tooth pulp and covered with enamel on the crown, and on the roots by cementum.

J

JACOBSON'S NERVE: (TYMPANIC NERVE) Ludwic L. Jacobson, Danish Physician. A branch of the glossopharyngeal (IX cranial) nerve serving sensory and parasynpathetic functions,distribution to the auditory tube, mastoid air cells, and the tympanic cavity (middle ear).

JAW BONE: (MANDIBLE) The largest and strongest bone of the face forming the lower jaw. Being horseshoe shaped, the body is the horizontal portion and the ramus the perpendicular portion. The border of the body contains the alveolar process for reception of the teeth. Each ramus has a condyloid process which forms the mandibular head, fitting into the mandibular fossa of the temporal bone. The coronoid process serves for the attachment of the temporalis muscle and some fibers of the buccinator muscle. Seperating the two processes is the mandibular notch. Between the lower and upper border of the body, at a point below the first molar tooth on each side, is the mental foramen the passage for the mental nerve, a branch of the trigeminal (V cranial) nerve. It articulates with the two temporal bones, contains the lower teeth, serves as points of attachment for the tongue and other muscles, and through movement, changes the acoustic characteristics and size of the oral cavity. pl. mandiblae.

JOINT: Point of contact between two bones formed by the cartilage and fibrous connective tissue. Joints are classified as: amphiarthrosis (slightly moveable), diarthrodial (freely moveable), and synarthrodial (immovable).

JOINT CAPSULE: Fibrous tissue coverning a joint.

JUGULAR: The neck region. 2. The large vein in the neck.

JUGULAR FORAMEN: The opening formed by the occipital and temporal bone jugular notches for passage of the accessory (XI cranial), glossopharyngeal (IX cranial), vagus (X cranial), and other arteries and veins.

JUGULAR FOSSA: A deep depression on the inferior surface of the temporal bone petrous portion. It forms the anterior and lateral wall of the jugular foramen, and a portion of the jugular notch.

JUGULAR GANGLIA: (SUPERIOR GANGLION) An enlargement of the vagus (X cranial) nerve in the jugular foramen from which motor and sensory fibers communicate with the accessory (XI cranial), Facial (VII cranial), and glossopharyngeal (IX cranial) nerves.

JUGULAR NOTCH: (SUPRASTERNAL NOTCH) The notch on the superior border of the sternum bone between the clavicular notches.

JUGULAR PROCESS- OCCOPITAL BONE: A projection of bone, from the occipital bone condyles, forming the jugular foramen posterior edge.

JUGULAR WALL:(FUNDUS TYMPANIC) A thin plate of bone that forms the floor of the tympanic cavity (middle ear), seperating the cavity from the groove containing the jugular vein.

K

K: Symbol for potassium. A metallic element of the alkali group, being a soft silver-white metal.

KARYOTHECA: Membrane inclosing a cell nucleus.

KINESTHESIA: Sense of movement of muscles, and the perception of position, resistance and weight.

KINETIC: Pertaining to motion.

KINOCILIUM: A thread-like filament on a cell surface which has spontaneous movement.

L

LABIA ORIS: The fleshy folds which form the opening of the mouth cavity, covered externally by skin and internally by mucous membrane. Between this coverning is fat, glandular tissue, nerves and the orbicularis oris muscle. The tissue of the lips is in four layers in order of depth; cutaneous, muscular, glandular, and mucous. On the inner surface, the upper lip connects to the alveolar process at midline by a fold of mucous membrane, the frenulum. A similar smaller frenulum connects the alveolar process of the mandible bone with the lower lip. The labial glands are pea-size, around the opening of the mouth between the mucous membrane and the orbicularis oris muscle.

LABIAL: Pertaining to the lips.

LABIAL FRENULUM INFERIOR: Fold of mucous membrane connecting at midline the inside of the lower lip with the gingiva (gums).

LABIAL FRENULUM SUPERIOR: Fold of mucous membrane connecting at midline the inside of the upper lip with the gingiva (gums).

LABIAL GLANDS: Located between the mucous membrane and the orbicularis oris muscle around the opening of the mouth. The glands are pea-shaped with ducts opening on the mucous membrane.

LABIODENTIAL: Pertaining to the lips and teeth.

LABIOVERSION: The displacement of a tooth tilted toward the lips.

LABIUM: A fleshy border, such as the lip.

LABYRINTH: The internal ear consisting of the membranous and osseous portions. 2. A portion of the ethmoid bone consisting of the thin walled cellular cavities and the ethmoidal cells. 3. A system of interconnecting pathways.

LABYRINTHIC: (MEDIAL WALL) The inner wall of the tympanic cavity (middle ear). Vertical in direction and containing the fenestra vestibuli (oval window), fenestra rotunda (round window), promontory and the prominence of the facial canal.

LABYRINTHINE ARTERY: (BASILAR ARTERY-INTERNAL AUDITORY) (COCHLEAR ARTERY) A branch of the basilar artery directed through the internal auditory canal to the inner ear.

LABYRINTHINE PRESSURE THEORY: Proposes that the tympanic musculature, by making various degrees of contraction, produces a change of air pressure of the inner ear or fluids. The increase in pressure produce an increase in mechanical resistance and a corresponding loss of low frequency transmission.

LACRIMAL BONE: The smallest, thinest most fragile bone of the face. Forms a portion of the orbital cavity medial wall. It contains the nasal and orbital surfaces and articulates with the ethmoid, frontal, inferior nasal concha, and maxilla bones.

LACRIMAL FOSSA: (LACRIMAL GROOVE) A groove formed by the lacrimal bone sulcus and the maxilla bone frontal process. At its superior part the lacrimal sac.

LACRIMAL NERVE: A sensory nerve, the smallest of the three branches of the ophthamic nerve, the first division of the trigeminal (V cranial) nerve, directed to the upper eyelid.

LACUNA: A cavity or pit. The space in the matrix or dense connective tissue occupied by a cartilage cell or by a bone cell. pl. lacunae.

LAMELLA: A thin leaf or plate. pl. lamellae.

LAMINA: Flat layer of bone or plate. pl. laminae.

LAMINOGRAPHY: Radiographs of a certain place or section of the body.

LANDMARK: A structure used as a reference point to establish the location of another point or structure.

LARYNGOPHARYNX: The lowest portion of the pharyngeal cavity. It is bounded by the hyoid bone down to the edge of the cricoid cartilage and continuous with the esophagus. It communicates with the larynx opening formed anteriorly by the epiglottis and laterally by the aryepiglottis folds.

LARYNGOSCOPE: Instrument for examination of the interior portion of the larynx.

LARYNGOSCOPY: Examination of the interior portion of the larynx.

LARYNX: A cartilaginous muscular structure covered with mucous membrane at the top of the trachea and below the hyoid bone and tongue. It is somewhat triangular shaped, formed by nine cartilages; cricoid, epiglottis, thyroid, and two of the arytenoid, corniculate and cuneiform which are connected by extrinsic and intrinsic ligaments. The larynx cavity is divided into two portions, infraglottal and supraglottal, by the true vocal folds. The two mucous membrane folds from back to front leave an elongated fissure, the glottis, which is protected by a lead-shaped, lid-like fibrocartilage, the epiglottis. The fissure contains fibrous and elastic ligaments giving its edge elasticity.

LARYNX-BIOLOGICAL FUNCTIONS: Acts as a valve by expelling by force foreign matter which threatens enterance into the trachea. Prevents air from escaping from the lunds, and prevents foreign matter from entering the trachea.

LARYNX CAVITY: Divided by the vocal folds from the laryngeal opening to the lower border of the cricoid cartilage. The cavity contains the true vocal folds (vocal cords) and the ventricular folds (false vocal folds).

LARYNX MEMBRANES-EXTRINSIC: Ligaments that connect the epiglottis and thyroid cartilage with the hyoid bone and the cricoid cartilage with the trachea; consists of the hyothyroid membrane, and cricotracheal, lateral hyothyoid and hyoepiglottic ligaments.

LARYNX MEMBRANES-INTRINSIC: Ligaments which connect several cartilages of the larynx to each other, the conus elasticus (crico-thyroid membrane) and the quadrangular membrane, aryepiglottic folds and the anterior and posterior cricoarytenoid ligaments.

LARYNX VESTIBULE: The area of the larynx cavity above the vocal folds. Triangular-shaped, being wider in front than behind.

LATENT PERIOD: The time between the instant of stimulus and the beginning of muscle contraction.

LATERAL: Away from the midline. Toward the external boundry or surface of the body.

LATERAL COLUMN: Consists of cell bodies of the sympathetic nervous system located in the lateral portion of the spinal cord gray matter.

LATERAL CORTICOSPHINAL TRACT: (LATERAL PYRAMIDAL TRACT) The descending motor tract for voluntary movement with distribution throughout the spinal cord.

LATERAL CRICOARYTENOID MUSCLE: (CRICOARYTENOID MUSCLE-LATERAL) A broad fan-shaped intrinsic adductor of the larynx. ORIGIN-The upper surface of the cricoid cartilage. DIRECTION- Upward and backward. INSERTION- Arytenoid cartilage muscular process. ACTION- Brings together the vocal folds. NERVE- Vagus (X cranial) laryngeal and recurrent branches.

LATERAL FISSURE: (FISSURE OF SYLVIUS)Francois Sylvius, French Anatomist. A fissure which seperates the temporal lobe from the frontal and parietal lobes of the brain. It begins at the inferior border and courses backward and up to terminate on the lateral surface.

LATERAL FUNICULUS-ASCENDING TRACTS: (SPINAL CORD LATERAL FUNICULUS-ASCENDING TRACTS) Consists of the dorsal spinocere-beller, dorsolateral, lateral proper fasciculus, lateral spinothalamic, spinotectal and ventral spinocerebeller tracts.

LATERAL FUNICULUS-DESCENDING TRACTS: (SPINAL CORD LATERAL FUNICULUS-DECENDING TRACTS) Consists of the lateral corticospinal, lateral reticulospinal, olivospinal and rubrospinal tracts.

LATERAL GENICULATE BODY: An elevation of the posterior end of the thalamus connected to the superior colliculus by the superior brachium.

LATERAL HYOTHYROID LIGAMENT: (THYROHYOID LIGAMENT) An extrinsic elastic cord-like ligament which syspends the larynx from the hyoid bone. The cord forms the posterior border of the hyo-thyroid membrane and extends from the posterior tip of the greater horn of the hyoid bone to the superior tip of the thyroid cartilage. A small cartilaginous nodule may be found imbedded in the ligament, the triticial cartilage.

LATERAL LEMNISCUS: A bundle of sensory fibers in the caudal por-tion of the midbrain, dorsal to the medial lemniscus. Responsible for the palpebroacoustic reflex (startle response). Along the path-way some auditory fibers are directed to the facial (VII cranial) nerve, while others terminate in the medial geniculate body.

LATERAL PTERYGOID NERVE: A motor nerve branch of the mandibular nerve. The third and largest division of the trigeminal (V cranial) nerve directed to the lateral pterygoid muscle.

LATERAL LIGAMENT: (TEMPOROMANDIBULAR LIGAMENT) Two short bundles from the lateral surface of the zygomatic arch to the lateral surface, posterior border, of the neck of the mandible bone condy-loid process.

LATERAL LIGAMENT OF THE MALLEUS BONE: (MALLEI LATERALE LIGA-MENT) A triangular shaped band from the notch of Rivinus to the head or neck of the malleus bone in the tympanic cavity (middle ear).

LATERAL MASS: (LABYRINTH) A portion of the ethmoid bone consist-ing of the ethmoidal cells, thin walled cellular cavities.

LATERAL NASAL: A portion of the septal cartilage of the nose, infer-ior to the nasal bone.

LATERAL PARTS- OCCIPITAL BONE: (PARS LATERALIS) Located at the sides of the magnum foramen. The condyles are on the under surface for articulation with the superior facets of the first cervical vertebra (atlas).

LATERAL PROCESS- MALLEUS BONE: A cone-shaped projection from the root of the manubrium process that is attached to the upper portion of the tympanic membrane (eardrum).

LATERAL PTERYGOID PLATE: A thin wide plate with the lateral surface forming a portion of the infratemporal fossa for attachment of the pterygoideus lateralis muscle. The medial surface forms a portion of the pterygoid fossa for attachment of the pterygoideus medialis muscle.

LATERAL PYRAMIDAL TRACT: (LATERAL CORTICOSPHINAL TRACT) The descending motor tract for voluntary movement with distribution throughout the spinal cord.

LATERAL RETICULOSPINAL TRACT: A descending tract of fibers originating in the reticular formation and directed throughout the brain stem.

LATERAL SPINOTHALAMIC TRACT: An ascending tract of the spinal cord. Arising through the lateral strand of the dorsal root and terminating at the thalamus, which carries impulses for pain and temperature.

LATERAL VENTRICLE: Consists of two cavities, left and right, with one located in each hemisphere under the corpus callosum, a mass of white fibers and separated from each other by the septum pellucidum, a thin double partition. The cavity contains spinal fluid with communication with the third ventricle accomplished through the foramen of Monro. The ventricle is bounded inferiorly by the thalamus and laterally by the caudate nucleus. Each lateral ventricle consists of a body and the interior, inferior and posterior cornu. The cavity is of the original embryo neural canal.

LATERAL WALL: (MEMBRANOUS WALL) Formed by the tympanic membrane (eardrum) which is held in place by a fibrocartilaginous ring incomplete at the top to form the notch of Rivinus.

LATISSIMUS DORSI MUSCLE: A muscle of inhalation and of the back forming a portion of the second muscle layer. ORIGIN- The thoracic vertebrae seven through twelve and the lumbar and sacral vertebrae. DIRECTION-Upward and lateral. INSERTION- Groove of the humerus bone. ACTION- Extend the arm and raise lower ribs. NERVE- Branchial plexus.

LAYER: A sheetlike, thin mass usually uniform in thickness.

LEMNISCUS: A band or ribbon. pl. lemnisci.

LENTICULAR: Pertaining to, or shaped like, a lens.

LENTICULAR PROCESS: A knob on the long limb of the incus (anvil) bone which articulates with the stapes (stirrup) bone in the tympanic cavity (middle ear).

LENTICULAR NUCLEUS: (LENIFORM NUCLEUS) A wedge-shaped mass of gray matter located lateral to the internal capsule. It forms a portion of the corpus striatum, divided into the globus pallidus and globus.

LESSER ALAR: (SESAMOID) The cartilage forming a portion of the lateral wall of the nose.

LESSER CORNU: The small horns of the hyoid bone, for attachment of the stylohyoid ligament.

LESSER PALATINE FORAMEN: (MINOR PALATINE FORAMEN) The opening in the palatine bone behind the palatine crest on the pyramidal process for passage of vessels.

LESSER PALATINE NERVES: Sensory branches of the pterygopalatine nerves, a branch of the maxillary nerve, the second division of the trigeninal (V cranial) nerve. Directed to the soft palate, tonsil, and uvula.

LEVATOR: That which raises or elevates.

LEVATOR ANGULI ORIS: (CANINE MUSCLE) A muscle of the mouth for facial expression. ORIGIN- Maxilla bone canine fossa. DIRECTION-Downward and oblique. INSERTION- Orbicularis oris muscle and the skin at the mouth angle. ACTION- Raises mouth angle. NERVE- Facial (VII cranial).

LEVATOR LABII SUPERIORIS MUSCLE:(QUADRATUS LABII SUPERIOR) A triangular muscle of the mouth above the upper lip with origin from three heads.
Angular head-ORIGIN- Maxilla bone frontal process. DIRECTION-Downward and lateral. INSERTION- Nostril cartilage and orbicularis oris muscle. ACTION- Raise upper lip, dilates the nostril. NERVE- Facial (VII cranial) buccal branch. Infraorbital head- ORIGIN Lower margin of the orbit. DIRECTION- Downward. INSERTION-Orbicularis oris muscle. ACTION- Raise upper lip. NERVE- Facial

(VII cranial) buccal branch. Zygomatic head- ORIGIN- Zygomatic bone, malar surface. DIRECTION- Downward and medial. INSERTION- Orbicularis oris muscle. ACTION- Raise upper lip. NERVE- Facial (VII franial) buccal branch.

LEVATOR PALATINE MUSCLE: (LEVATOR VELI PALATINE MUSCLE: A muscle of the soft palate located lateral to the nasal choanae. ORI ORIGIN- Temporal bone petrous portion near the apex and cartilage of the auditory tube. DIRECTION- Downward and medial. INSERTION: Aponeurosis of the soft palate. ACTION: Raises soft palate. NERVE- Vagus (X cranial) Pharyngeal plexus.

LEVATORES COSTARUM: A muscle of the thorax in two groups. The levatores costarum brevis and levatores costarum longus.

Costarum brevis: ORIGIN - From the seventh cervical and next eleven thoracic vertebrae. DIRECTION-Downward and lateral. INSERTION- Outer surface of the ribs under the points of origin. ACTION- Flex vertebral column, raise ribs. NERVE- Intercostal nerve branches. Costarum lonus: ORIGIN- From the seventh cervical and next eleven thoracic vertebrae. DIRECTION-Rib under the point of origin. INSERTION- Outer surface of the second rib below the point of origin. ACTION- Flex vertebral column, raise ribs. NERVE- Intercostal nerve branches.

LEVER SYSTEM: The human skeletal system contains three lever systems: Class I- Operates with a mechanical advantage or disadvantage. Many muscles are part of the system with a disadvantage. Power is lost for increased speed of movement. Class II- Operates with a mechanical advantage. Opening the jaw against an opposing force is an example. Class III- Operates with a mechanical disadvantage. Although power is lost, rapid movement is gained.

LIGAMENT: A sheet of strong elastic fibrous connective tissue that attaches bone to bone, bone to cartilage, or cartilage to cartilage.

LIGAMENTS OF THE OSSICULAR CHAIN: The ossicles of the tympanic cavity (middle ear) are connected to the walls and supported by the posterior ligament for the incus (anvil) bone, the anterior, lateral, and superior ligaments for the malleus (hammer) bone; the annular ligament for the stapes (stirrup) bone.

LIMBUS: The border or fringe of an organ or structure. pl. limbi.

LIMITANS: Used with other descriptive words to state borders. 2. To indicate membranous limits.

LINE: A mark, narrow ridge, streak, or stripe on the surface of a structure.

LINEA ALBA: (WHITE LINE) A fibrous dense white band of tissue at midline extending from the ensiform porcess of the sternum bone to the pubic symphysis, for the attachment of the abdominal oblique and transverse muscles.

LINEA SEMILUNARIS: Two layers of tendon, lateral to the rectus abdominis muscle. It divides into three layers of aponeourosis which serve for the insertion of the lateral abdominal muscles. The upper layer attaches superiorly to the bottom fibers of the pectoralis major muscle, the sternum bone ensiform process and costal cartilages.

LINGUA: A shape simular to a tongue. 2. A moveable muscular organ on the floor of the mouth. pl. linguae.

LINGUA: (TONGUE) The organ of the mouth attached by mucous membrane to the floor of the mouth and by muscles to the epiglottis, hyoid bone, mandible bone, palate, pharynx walls and styloid process. It is free to move anteriorly, dorsally and laterally aiding in degulition, mastication and in speech production. Its movement modifies the resonance characteristics of the oral cavity and in the production of voiced consonants. The tongue is divided anatomically into the blade and root; functionally into the back, blade, front and tip. The surface contains papillae of three types, filiform, fungiform and vallate.

LINGUA FRENULUM: The membrane extending from the interior surface of the tongue to the mouth floor. pl. linguae.

LINGUAL GYRUS: A convolution located on the inferior surface of the occipital lobe.

LINGUAL NERVE: A sensory nerve branch of the mandibular nerve, the third and largest division of the trigeminal (V cranial) nerve. It further divides into branches directed to the chorda tympani and hypoglossal nerves, and the mucous membrane of the gums, mouth and the tongue anterior portion.

LINGUAL NERVE BRANCHES: Sensory branchs of the glossopharyn-geal (IX cranial) nerve directed to the glands and mucous membrane of the tongue.

LINGUAL PAPILLA: Either of the filiform, fungiform, and conical papillae covering the tongue.

LINGUAL SEPTUM: A sheet of connective tissue which separates the tongue into halves.

LINGUAL TONSIL: A mass of lymhoid tissue forming the anterior por-tion of the tonsil ring. Located in the tonsillar fossa, which is form-ed by the palatoglossal and palatopharyngeal arches.

LINGULA: A structure that is tongue-like.

LINGULA OF THE CEREBELLUM: The point on the cerebellum ventral surface for attachment of the superior medullary velum.

LINGUOVERSION: The displacement of a tooth tilted toward the tongue.

LIPS: (LABIA ORIS) The fleshy folds which form the opening of the mouth cavity, covered externally by skin and internally by mucous membrane. Between this coverning is fat, glandular tissue, nerves and the orbicularis oris muscle. The tissue of the lips is in four layers in order of depth; cutaneous, muscular, glandular and muc-ous. On the inner surface, the upper lip connects to the alveolar process at midline by a fold of mucous membrane, the frenulum. A similar smaller frenulum connects the alveolar process of the mandible cone with the lower lip. The labial glands are pea-size, around the opening of the mouth between the mucous membrane and the orbicularis oris muscle.

LIPID: Fat, or fat-like substance, that is insoluble in water.

LIP-TEETH (LABIODENTAL) Pertaining to the llips and teeth. 2. A consonant classification of articulators used and the position they are in.

LOBE: A well defined portion of an organ.

LOBULE: A small lobe.

LOGARITHM: The small number, the exponent placed higher and to the right of the base number to indicate the base number must be raised to that power to produce a given number. The logarithm or exponent numbers are determined through the use of logarithm tables. The decibel (dB) is a unit of measurement to express a ratio to the base 10.

LONG CRUS: (LONG PROCESS)- INCUS BONE: Descends downward, behind and parallel to the manubrium process of the malleus (hammer) bone and ends as a round projection, the lenticular process which articulates with the stapes (stirrup) bone head.

LONGITUDINAL: Lengthwise, or in the direction of the long axis of the body.

LONGITUDINAL FISSURE: The deep fissure at midline between the two cerebral hemispheres.

LONGUS: Long.

LOOSE TEETH: Gomphiasis.

LOUDNESS: The intensity of a sound, dependent upon the frequency.

LOWER JAW: (MANDIBLE BONE) The largest and strongest bone of the face forming the lower jaw. Being horseshoe shaped, the body is the horizontal portion and the ramus the perpendicular portion. The border of the body contains the alveolar process for reception of the teeth. Each ramus has a condyloid process which forms the mandibular head, fitting into the mandibular fossa of the temporal bone. The coronoid process serves for the attachment of the temporalis muscle and some fibers of the buccinator muscle. Seperating the two processes is the mandibular notch. Between the lower and upper border of the body, at a point below the first molar tooth on each side, is the mental foramen for passage of the mental nerve, a branch of the trigeminal (V cranial) nerve. It articulates with the two temporal bones, contains the lower teeth, serves as points of attachment for the tongue and other muscles, and through movement, changes the acoustic characteristics and size of the oral cavity. pl. mandiblae.

LOW PASS FILTER: A device, electrical, or mechanical which attenuates high frequency energy and passes the low frequency energy.

LUMBAR: Portion of the back between the thorax and the pelvis.

LUMBAR APONEUROSIS: A superficial aponeurosis at the origin of

the transversus abdominis muscle. Along with the lumbocostal
aponeurosis it encloses the sacrosponalis muscle.

LUMBAR FASCIA: A broad sheet of tendon on the dorsal portion of
the lower vertebral column. It attaches on the posterior portion
of the iliac crest and lumbar vertebrae spines. It further divides
into two layers of aponeurosis into which muscle fibers from the
internal oblique and transverseus abdominis muscles insert.

LUMBAR NERVES: Five pair of nerves in the lumbar area arising
from the lumbar segments of the spinal cord.

LUMBAR PLEXUS: A network of nerves formed by the four pair of
lumbar nerves.

LUMBAR VERTEBRA: Five bones of the spinal column between the
sacrum and thoracic vertebrae.

LUMBOSACRAL PLEXUS: The network of the ventral primary divisions
of the coccygeal, lumbar, and sacral nerves which communicate to
the lower limbs and trunk.

LUMEN: Cavity or channel within a tube. pl. lumina.

LUNG: One of two cone-shaped, irregular, porous, spongy, highly
elastic, organs of respiration within the pleural cavity of the thorax.
The apex extends past the thorax into the neck above the superior
border of the first rib. The base conforms to the superior surface
of the diaphragm, being concave shaped. The diaphragm separates
the left lung base from the liver, spleen, and stomach; the right
lung from a major portion of the liver. Each lung has an anterior,
inferior, and posterior border. The anterior border separates the
mediastinal surface from the costal surface. The inferior border is
the division between the back, mediastinal, and thoracic surfaces.
The posterior border separates, by an undifined line, the mediastinal surface from the costal surface. The lung capacity of an adult
male is approximately five thousand cubic centimeters of air. In
shape the right lung is broader, larger and shorter than the left.
The left lung is divided by an oblique fissure into the inferior and
superior lobe, with an indentation for the normal place of the
heart, the cardiac depression. The right lung is divided into three
lobes by two fissures. The horizontal fissure divides the middle
small lobe. The oblique fissure separates the inferior and superior
lobe.

LYMPH; Fluid secreted by the lymph glands in order to expedite the removal of waste from tissue cells.

M

MACULA: An area that is different in color than its surroundings. 2. A spot or stain. pl. maculae.

MACULA ACUSTICAE: The thickened areas of the saccule and utricle where the termination of the vestibular branch of the auditory (VIII cranial) nerve occurs. These areas are sensory and contain hair cells which respond to fluid movement.

MACULA ACUSTICA SACCULI: A thickened area in the anterior portion of the saccule containing fibers of the auditory (VIII cranial) nerve.

MACULA ACUSTICA UTRICULI: A thickened area in the floor and wall of the utricle containing fibers of the auditory (VIII cranial) nerve.

MAGMA RETICULARE: In embryo development, the developing mesoderm within the chorionic sac.

MAJOR PALATINE FORAMEN: (GREATER PALATINE FORAMEN) The opening at either posterior angle of the hard palate for passage of the palatine nerve.

MALA: The cheek or cheekbone.

MALAR: Pertaining to the cheek or cheekbone.

MALAR BONE: (CHEEK BONE) (ZYGOMATIC BONE) Located at the lateral and upper portion of the face. Quadrangular in shape with processes of frontosphenoidal, maxillary, orbital and temporal, and the malar (outer) and temporal surfaces. It forms along with the zygomatic process of the maxilla and temporal bones, the zygomatic arch (cheek bone) and a portion of the orbital cavity lateral floor and wall. It articulates with the frontal, maxilla, spenoid and temporal bones.

MALAR SURFACE- ZYGOMATIC BONE: A convex surface with an opening near the center (zygomaticofacial foramen) for passage of the zygomaticofacial nerve and vessels.

MALLEI ANTERIOR LIGAMENT: (ANTERIOR LIGAMENT OF THE MALLEUS BONE) A band of fiber, one end attached to the malleus (hammer) bone neck, with the other end attached to the tympanic cavity (middle ear) anterior wall.

MALLEI CAPITULUM: (HEAD OF MALLEUS) The superior portion of the malleus bone containing the facet for articulation by a diarthrodial joint with the incus (anvil) bone.

MALLEI LATERALE LIGAMENT: (LATERAL LIGAMENT OF THE MALLEUS BONE) A triangular shaped band from the notch of Rivinus to the malleus (hammer) bone head or neck.

MALLEI SUPERIOR LIGAMENT: (SUPERIOR LIGAMENT OF THE MALLEUS BONE) A thin strand desending from the roof of the tympanic cavity (middle ear) to the malleus (hammer) bone head.

MALLEOINCUDAL JOINT: A enarthrosis (ball and socket) type joint with a articular disc encircled by an articular capsule.

MALLEOLAR FOLDS: The anterior and superior folds of tissue which mark the line between the pars flaccida and pars tensa portions of the tympanic membrane (eardrum). The anterior fold covers a portion of the chorda tympanic nerve, a portion of the facial (VII cranial) nerve.

MALLEOLAR STRIA: A vertical whitish streak on the outer surface of the tympanic membrane (eardrum) directed from the umbo upward. It is caused by the attachment of the manubrium (handle) of the malleus (hammer) bone to the eardrum.

MALLEUS BONE: (HAMMER) The first and largest ossicle attached to the tympanic membrane (eardrum), and to the incus (anvil) bone by a diarthrodial joint. It consist of the head, neck, the anterior, lateral and manubrium processes.

MALLEUS HEAD: The oval shaped portion of the malleus (hammer) bone containing a articular facet for articulating with the incus (anvil) bone. The lower margin of the facet extends to form a cog tooth process.

MALLEUS NECK: A narrow contracted area between the head and manubrium process of the malleus (hammer) bone.

MALOCCLUSION: Any deviation from the normal closure of the teeth.

MAMMILLARY BODIES: Two round-like, gray masses on each side of midline near the cerebral peduncles forming a portion of the hypothalamus.

MANDIBLE BONE: (LOWER JAW) The largest and strongest bone of the face forming the lower jaw. Being horseshow shaped, the body is the horizontal portion and the ramus the perpendicular portion. The border of the body contains the alveolar process for reception of the teeth. Each ramus has a condyloid process which forms the mandibular head, fitting into the mandibular fossa of the temporal bone. The coronoid process serves for the attachment of the temporalis muscle and some fibers of the buccinator muscle. Separating the two processes is the mandibular notch. Between the lower and upper border of the body, at a point below the first molar tooth on each side, is the mental foramen for passage of the mental nerve, a branch of the trigeminal (V cranial) nerve. It articulates with the two temporal bones, contains the lower teeth, serves as points of attachment for the tongue and other muscles, and through movement, changes the acoustic characteristics and size of the oral cavity. pl. mandiblae.

MANDIBULAR ARCH: The first branchial arch in embryo development from which the lower and upper jaw bone, and incus and malleus bones develop.

MANDIBULAR CANAL: A canal in the mandible bone for passage of the alveolar vessels and nerves to the teeth.

MANDIBULAR FORAMEN: The opening on the medial surface of the mandible bone into the mandibular canal for passage of the inferior alveolar nerve, a branch of the mandibular nerve, the third and largest division of the trigeminal (V cranial) nerve.

MANDIBULAR FOSSA: (GLENOID FOSSA) A depression in the surface of the squama portion of the temporal bone at the base of the zygomatic process in which the mandible bone condyloid process rest.

MANDIBULAR NERVE: A motor and sensory nerve, the third and largest division of the trigeminal (V cranial) nerve. The anterior motor portion is directed to the muscles of mastication, and the posterior portion is directed to the external ear, cheek, lower lip, lower portion of the face, gums and teeth, tongue and skin of the temporal area.

MANDIBULAR NERVE BRANCH; A motor branch of the facial (VII cranial) nerve directed to the chin and lower lip.

MANDIBULAR NOTCH: (SEMILUNAR NOTCH) A deep depression on the mandible bone ramus portion on the superior border separating the coronoid and condyloid processes.

MANOMETER: Device for measuring gas or liquid pressure.

MANTLE: A coverning or layer.

MANTLE LAYER: (MANTLE ZONE) In embryo development, the middle layer of the three layer primitive neural tube. Consisting of germinal cells which develop into nerve cells of the central nervous system and spongioblasts which develop into supporting neuroglia.

MANUBRIUM: The superior portion of the sternum bone which articulates with the clavicle bone and first pair of costal cartilages. 2. Handle shaped. pl. manubria.

MANUBRIUM PROCESS-MALLEUS BONE: Long and narrow, directed backward, downward, and medially. A projection forming a point where the tensor tympani muscle attaches.

MARGIN: (MARGO) The border, or edge of an organ or structure.

MARGINAL LAYER: (MARGINAL ZONE) In embryo development, the outer layer of the three layer primitive neural tube. Consisting of a fibrous mesh-like layer forming the white substance of the central nervous system.

MARROW: (BONE MARROW) The soft material filling the cavities of spongy bone. It consist of red marrow which produces red blood cells and is found in flat and short bones such as ribs, sternum and vertebrae bodies. Yellow marrow, which is fat cells is found in the large cavities of long bones in the arms and legs.

MASS: A body or lump made up of cohering particles. pl. massae.

MASSETER MUSCLE: A strong thick muscle of mastication. ORIGIN-From two layers: Deep layer- Posterior surface of the zygomatic arch. Superficial layer- Lower border of the zygomatic arch.

DIRECTION- Deep- Downward and forward. Superficial- Downward and backward. INSERTION- Deep Mandible bone superior ramus and coronoid process. Superficial- Mandible bone ramus and lateral surface. ACTION- Closes jaws, raises mandible bone. NERVE- Trigeminal (V cranial) mandibular division.

MASSETERIC NERVE: A motor and sensory branch of the mandibular nerve, the third and largest division of the trigeminal (V cranial) nerve directed to the masseter muscle and temporomandibular joint.

MASTICATION: Chewing of food.

MASTICATION MUSCLES: Consist of the digastricus, external ptery- goid, internal pterygoid, geniohyoid, and mylohyoid muscles.

MASTOID: Nipple-shaped. 2. The mastoid process of the temporal bone.

MASTOID AIR CELLS: Found in the mastoid process of the tomporal bone and vary in number and size. At the front and upper portion they are irregular, large, and contain air, but decrease in size toward the lower portion.

MASTOID ANTRUM:(TYMPANIC ANTRUM) A air filled, mucous mem- brane lined cavity anterior and superior to the mastoid process of the temporal bone. It communicates with the mastoid air cells and tympanic cavity (middle ear). The cavity is bounded by the tegmen above, mastoid process below, and squama portion of the temporal bone laterally and medially.

MASTOID NOTCH: A deep groove on the medial side of the temporal bone mastoid portion for the insertion of the digastricus muscle.

MASTOID PORTION-TEMPORAL BONE: Forms the posterior portion of the temporal bone and the mastoid process, a conical projection of the témporal bone. The process contains a number of small spaces, the mastoid air cells. Located anterior and superior to the process is another air filled cavity, the tympanic antrum which communi- cates with the mastoid air cells and tympanic cavity (middle ear).

MASTOID PROCESS: A conical projection on the mastoid portion of the temporal bone contaning numerous air spaces, the mastoid air cells.

MASTOID WALL: (POSTERIOR WALL) Forms the posterior portion of the the tympanic cavity (middle ear), and is wider above than below. It contains the enterance to the tympanic antrum, pyramidal eminence and fossa incudis.

MATRIX: Cavity in which anything is formed. Ground substance of connective tissue. pl. matrices.

MAXILLA BONE: (UPPER JAW BONE) The second largest facial bone. It is a paired bone forming the total upper jaw, a majority of the floor and lateral walls of the nasal cavity, the roof of the mouth. Each bone consists of a pyramidal shaped body containing the maxillary sinus and alveolar, frontal, palatine, and zygomatic processes. Each bone articulates with the frontal and ethmoid bones of the cranium and the inferior nasal conchea, lacimal, nasal, palatine, and zygomatic bones of the face. pl. maxillae.

MAXILLA BONE-FRONTAL PROCESS: (NASAL PROCESS) A stong boney plate directed upward, medial, and posteriorly. Forms the lateral frame of the nose, and the medial surface contributing to the lateral wall of the nasal cavity.

MAXILLARY NERVE: A sensory nerve, the second of three divisions of the trigeminal (V cranial) nerve. It divides into the anterior superior alveolar, external nasal, inferior palpebral, middle meningeal, middle superior alveolar, posterior superior alveolar, pterygopalatine, superior labial, and zygomatic branches. These in turn supply the cheek, hard palate, maxillary sinuses, nasal mucous, upper jaw, and teeth with the sensation of pain and touch.

MAXILLARY PROCESS- INFERIOR NASAL CONCHA: On the lateral surface curving down and laterally forming a portion of the maxillary sinus medial wall and articulating with the maxilla bone.

MAXILLARY PROCESS- ZYGOMATIC BONE: A rough triangle-shaped surface which articulates with the maxilla bone.

MAXILLARY SINUS: (ANTRUM OF HIGHMORE) A large pyramid shaped cavity in the maxilla bone body. The apex extends into the zygomatic process and the base is formed by the nasal cavity lateral wall. It communicates with the middle passage of the nasal cavity on the same side. They appear from the fourth month of fetal life and are developed fully by puberty.

MAXILLARY TUBEROSITY: A round eminence on the infratemporal surface of the maxilla bone which articulates with the palatine bone.

MAXIMUM MINUTE BREATHING: (MAXIMUM MINUTE VOLUME) The

quantity of air exchange in a minute, with forced breathing.

MEATUS: A canal or passage.

MEATUS ACUSTICUS EXTERNUS: The portion of the external ear canal, consisting of cartilage from the outer ear to the bony portion of the canal which ends at the tympanic membrane (eardrum).

MECKEL'S CARTILAGE: Johann F. Meckel, Berlin Anatomist. In embryo development, the cartilage of the first branchial arch.

MEDIAL: (MESIAL) In the middle. Toward the midline.

MEDIAL GENICULATE BODY: A small tubercle at the posterior of the thalamus. Acts as a relay between the auditory center and inferior colliculus.

MEDIAN LINE: An imaginary line passing through the center of the body.

MEDIAL PTERYGOID NERVE: A motor nerve of the mandibular nerve, the third and largest division of the trigeminal (V cranial) nerve. Directed to the medial pterygoid muscle and further branches to the tensor tympani and tensor veli palatine muscles.

MEDIAL PTERYGOID PLATE: A long thin plate curved at the end into a hook-like process, the hamulus, around which the tensor veli palatine muscle moves.

MEDIAL RAPHE: (PALATINE RAPHE) A faint line or ridge in the midline of the palate.

MEDIAL WALL: (LABYRINTHIC) Forms the medial wall of the tympanic cavity (middle ear). Vertical in direction it contains the fenestra vestibuli (oval window), fenestra rotunda (round window), promontory, and prominence of the facial canal.

MEDIAL SULCUS: A slight depression on the dorsum of the tongue at midline. Ends near the tongue root in a depression, the foramen cecum.

MEDIASTINUM:The space in the center area of the thorax. Its boundary is on each side of a lung and pleural sac. It is divided into; anterior-containing lymph nodes; middle- containing the heart, which is enclosed by the pericardium; posterior- containing the greater blood vessels and a portion of the esophagus. and superior-containing blood vessels which supply the heart, part of the eso-phagus, and trachea, and nerves. 2. A cavity or septum between two portions of an organ. pl. mediastina.

MEDIUM: Substance that communicates impulses. pl. media.

MEDULLA: The middle. 2. The inner portion of an organ or structure. pl. medullae.

MEDULLA OBLONGATA: The most inferior and uppermost portion of the brain and spinal cord. It connects with the pons and contains motor nuclei of the glossopharyngeal (IX cranial), vagus (X cranial) accessory (XI cranial) and hypoglossal (XII cranial) nerves.

MEDULLARY FOLD: (NEURAL FOLD) In embryo development, two folds, one on each side of the neural plate. In the third and fourth week, the folds join each other to form the neural tube.

MEDULLARY LAMINA: Layers of white fibers over the surface of the thalamus.

MEDULLARY PLATE: (NEURAL PLATE) In embryo development, a plate of thickened ectoderm, the origin of the central nervous system, with the caudal portion forming the spinal cord and the rostral end forming the brain.

MEDULLARY SHEATH: (SHEATH OF SCHWANN) Theodor Schwann, German Physician. A layer of myelin which surrounds nerve fibers and functions as an insulator.

MEDULLARY VELUM: (SUPERIOR MEDULLARY VELUM) A layer of fibers forming a portion of the fourth ventricle roof.

MEDULLOBLAST: A cell that can develop into a nuroblast, a nerve cell or spongiblast, which develops from the embryo neural tube.

MEIOSIS: Special process of cell division. It occurs in the matura-tion of sex cells. Each female nucleus receives one half of the chromosome characteristic of the somatic cells.

MELANIN: The dark pigment of the choroid of the eye, hair, skin, and substantia niga of the brain.

MEMBRANE: A thin layer of tissue that binds structures, lines cavities, or separates organs.

MEMBRANIFORM: Membrane-like.

MEMBRANE THEORY: Proposes a cell is surrounded by a membrane separating a double layer of ions, with negative ions inside and positive ions outside. The negative and positive charges are stable at rest. If a cell is disturbed a rapid ion exchange is made and the electrical charge changes.

MEMBRANOUS COCHLEA: (COCHLEA DUCT) (SCALA MEDIA) The tube triangular shaped within the cochlea separated from the scala vestibuii by Reissner's membrane and from the scala tympani by the basilar membrane. The duct contains the organ of Corti and endolymph fluid.

MEMBRANOUS GLOTTIS: (VOCAL GLOTTIS) The approximate anterior three-fifths of the rima glottis. Bounded laterally by the muscular portion of the true vocal folds it extends from the anterior commissure of the true vocal fold to the vocal process of the arytenoid cartilage.

MEMBRANOUS LABYRINTH: Simular in shape as the bony labyrinth and located within it, filled with endolymph fluid. At some areas it is adheared to the walls of the bony labryinth by connective tissue. It has three portions, cochlea duct, saccule and utricle, and the semicircular canals.

MEMBRANOUS WALL: (LATERAL WALL) Formed by the tympanic membrane (eardrum) held in place by a fibrocartilaginous ring incomplete at the top to form the notch of Rivinus.

MENINGES: Three layers of membranous tissue coverning the brain and spinal cord; outer layer, the dura mater; middle layer, the arachnoid; internal layer, the pia mater.

MENINX: One of the three membranes enclosing the brain and spinal ford. 2. A membrane. pl. meninges.

MENISCUS: A crescent shaped structure. pl. menisci.

MENTAL: The mind or chin.

MENTAL FORAMEN: A opening in the mandible bone, on each side midway between the lower and upper borders of the body, used for the passage of the mental nerve and blood vessels from the interior to the exterior surface.

MENTAL NERVE: A seonsory branch of the inferior alveolar nerve, a branch of the maxillary nerve, the third and largest division of the trigeminal (V cranial) nerve directed to the chin and lower lip.

MENTAL PROTUBERANCE: (CHIN) (POINT OF THE CHIN) A triangular projection formed by the dividing of the midline ridge (mental symphysis) near the lower border of the mandible bone.

MENTAL SPINES: Two small ridges, directed laterally, on the inner surface of the mandible bone near the midline mental symphysis.

MENTAL SYMPHYSIS: Point where the two halves of the mandible bone join and ossify during the first year forming a vertical midline ridge.

MENTAL TUBERCLES: Two anterior projections formed by the depression in the center of the triangular-shaped mental protuberance on the mandible bone.

MENTAL MUSCLE: (MENTALIS MUSCLE) A muscle of the mouth for facial expression. ORIGIN- Mandible bone incisive fossa. DIRECTION- Upward. INSERTION- Skin of the chin. ACTION- Raise skin and lower lip. NERVE- Facial (VII cranial) mandibular division.

MERCURY: A metallic element, liquid at ordinary temperature.

MESIAL: (MEDIAL) In the middle. Toward the midline.

MESENCEPHALON: (MIDBRAIN) The second of the three primary cerebral vesicles. From these are developed the corpora quadrigeminal (inferior and superior colliculi), cerebral aqueduct (of Sylvius), and crura cerebri in embryo development.

MESENCHYME: In embryo development, the connective tissue of the embryo. Part of the mesoderm, it forms the connective tissue and the blood vessels.

MESETHMOID: The perpendicular or vertical plate decending from the under surface of the cribform plate of the ethmoid bone.

MESIOCLUSION: In Angle's classification system, Class III, a protuded mandible bone in relation to the maxilla bone.

MESIOVERSION: The displacement of the anterior teeth tilted toward midline, or the posterior teeth tilted forward.

MESODERM: (DEFINITIVE MESODERM) In embryo development, the middle layer between the ectoderm and entoderm layers of the primary germ layers from which blood, blood vessels, bone, cartilage, and connective tissue are derived.

MESOPHRYON: (GLABELLA) The central point in the smooth area between the eyebrows.

MESOTENDON: The fibrous sheath of connective tissue connecting a tendon to its sheath.

MESOTHELIAL TISSUE: Composed of a sheet of areolar (connective) tissue covered with a layer of squamous (flat) cells. A special form of epithelid tissue, refered as serous membrane, which lines the body cavities.

MESOTHELIUM: A layer of flat cells which line the body cavity of the embryo.

METABOLISM: The total chemical and physical changes that occur in an organism.

METAPHASE: The second phase in mitosis (cell division), between prophase and anaphase, when the paired chromatids (chromosomes) are arranged between the centrioles to form the equatorial plate.

METATHALAMUS: The posterior portion of the thalamus, composed of the lateral and medial geniculate bodies.

METENCEPHALON: In embryo development, the anterior portion of the rhombencephalon (hindbrain). Formed by the development of the neural tube into a fold, which divides into two portions from which th4 cerebellum and pons develop.

METOPIC: Pertaining to the forehead.

METOPIC SUTURE: A union of the squama portion of the frontal bone which forms the forehead. At birth the bone is divided at midline, later joining and not usually present in adult life.

MICROBAR: (DYNE PER SQUARE CENTIMETER)(dyne/cm^2) A unit of measurement of sound pressure. The amount of energy necessary to accelerate one gram of material one centimeter per second per second.

MICROELECTRODE: A very small sensor used to contact a single cell.

MICRON: One-thousandth of a millimeter, 10^3 or one millionth of a meter, 10^3. Abbreviation, μ.

MICROPHONICS: An electrical noise signal generated by mechanical methods.

MICROSCOPE: Optical device that permits examination of minute objects.

MIDBRAIN: (MESENCPHALON) The second of the three primary cerebral vesicles. From these are developed the corpora quadrigeminal (inferior and superior colliculi), cerebral aqueduct (of Sylvius), and crura cerebri in embryo development.

MIDDLE CEREBELLAR PEDUNCLE: (BRACHIUM PONTIS) An area of the internal cerebellum which contains, on each side, fibers of the pons.

MIDDLE CONSTRICTOR: (CONSTRICTOR PHARYNGIS MEDIUS MUSCLE) A fan-shaped muscle of the pharynx. ORIGIN- From the hyoid bone greater and lesser cornu. DIRECTION- Fanning out backward and medial. INSERTION- On the medial raphe of the posterior wall of the pharynx. ACTION- Constricts the pharynx. NERVE- Glossopharyngeal (IX cranial) and vagus (X cranial) pharyngeal plexus.

MIDDLE EAR: (TYMPANIC CAVITY) A small irregular cavity in the temporal bone petrous portion. Contains the tympanic membrane (eardrum), the three bones of the ossicular chain, the incus (anvil), malleus (hammer), and stapes (stirrup), the fenestra rotunda (round window), fenestra vestibuli (oval window), and auditory (Eustachian) tube.

MIDDLE FRONTAL GYRUS: The convolution on the frontal lobe between the inferior and superior sulci, and divided by a longitudinal and middle frontal sulcus.

MIDDLE HYOTHYROID MEMBRANE: The thicker middle portion of the fibroelastic sheet, arising from the superior border of the thyroid cartilage. It has fibers directed upward to insert on the posterior surface of the body and greater cornu (horn) of the hyoid bone.

MIDDLE MENINGEAL NERVE: A sensory branch of the maxillary

nerve, the second division of the trigeminal (V cranial) nerve, directed to the dura mater.

MIDDLE NASAL CONCHA: The lower of two bony plates which project from the inner wall of the ethmoid labyrinth. Also separates the superior concha from the middle passage of the nose.

MIDDLE SUPERIOR ALVEOLAR NERVE BRANCH: A sensory branch of the maxillary nerve, the second division of the trigeminal (V cranial) nerve, directed to the premolar teeth and the superior dental plexes.

MIDDLE TEMPORAL GYRUS: The gyrus between the inferior and superior temporal sulci of the temporal lobe.

MIDGUT: In embryo development, the area opening into the yolk sac between the foregut and hindgut.

MIDSAGITTAL: An anatomic plane, from front to back, dividing into right and left parts.

MILK TEETH: The deciduous or first set of teeth .

MILLIMETER: One thousandth of a meter or approximately 0. 03937 inch (10^{-3}) Abbreviated; mm.

MINOR: Lesser or smaller.

MINOR PALATINE FORAMENT: (LESSER PALATINE FORAMEN) The opening in the palatine bone, behind the palatine crest on the pyramidal process, for passage of vessels.

MINUTE VOLUME; The total amount of air exchanged in one minute. Expressed as cm^2.

MITOCHONDRIA: (CHONDROSOMES) Highly complex structures with a smooth outer membrane and a variable folded inner membrane. The inner membrane may consists fo several extensions, which are shelf-like ridges in concentric layers, tubular or both. It is believed that they generate the power for cellular work through their chemical and respiratory functions. They are the "power plants of cells".

MITOSIS: Method of indirect division of a cell. pl. mitoses.

MITOSIS CELL DIVISION; The division of a cell. Divided into four phases; prophase, metaphase, anaphase, and telophase.

MIXED NERVE: A nerve consisting of both motor (efferent) and sensory (afferent) fibers.

mm: Abbreviation for millimeter, one thousandth of a meter or approximately 0. 03937 inch (10^{-3}).

MODALITY: A special sense such as sight or hearing.

MODULATE: To modify the frequency, intensity, or quality of the voice as in inflection or vibrato.

MOLAR TEETH: The posterior teeth on each jaw, eight in the deciduous and twelve in the permanent set. The crown is broad and square, used for grinding. The lower molars have two roots, the upper has three roots. The third molar (wisdom tooth) has roots fused together. The approximate eruption time as follows:

Deciduous- 1st molar 12-15 months Permanent- 1st 6-7 years
           2nd molar 24-40 months   2nd 12-15 years
                                             3rd 17-25 years

MOLAR GLANDS: Glands, smaller than the labial glands, located between the facial muscles and the mucous membrane of the cheek cheeks. Some of these, larger than others, opposite the last molar tooth open by ducts into the buccal cavity.

MOLECULAR LAYER OF CEREBELLUM: The outer layer of the cortex containing granular cells, horizontal cells of Cajal, and neuroglial cells.

MONAURAL: A single ear.

MORPHOLOGY: The study of form and structure.

MORULA: A mass of cells formed by a fertilized ovum.

MOSSY CELL: A non-nerve cell having a large body and several short processes.

MOTHER CELL: A cell which divides into two or more cells.

MOTOR: A center, muscle, or nerve that effects or produces movement.

MOTOR AREA: (AREA 4) The area of motor impulses anterior to the frontal lobe central sulcus forming a band from the lateral fissure to the dirsal border of the hemisphere. The left portion of the band

controls body right side action with the larynx and tongue controlled by the lower portion of the band.

MOTOR END PLATE: An expansion of a nerve termination where there
is no sheath around the nerve, ending in many small root-like
branches.

MOTOR FIBERS: Fibers of a mixed nerve which transmit only motor
impulses.

MOTOR NERVE: (MOTOR NEURON) Efferent nerve cell which excites a
muscular reaction.

MOTOR ROOT: (VENTRAL ROOT) Originates from within the gray
matter of the ventral columns of the spinal cord. Composed of
motor fibers which form two bundles near the intervertebral foramen, and transmits motor impulses from the spinal cord to the
periphery.

MOTOR UNIT: A functional unit for producing muscle action. Consisting of a nerve cell body, its processes, and muscle fiber. It may
consist of from a few, to a hundred or more muscle fibers.

MOUTH; The opening of a cavity. 2. The buccal cavity.

MOUTH CAVITY: (BUCCAL CAVITY) Consists of the vestibule, with
external boundries of the cheeks, lips, and mouth cavity proper
with internal boundries of the gingivae (gums) and teeth. Its shape
and size depend on the structure of the cheeks and lips.

MUCIN: A glycoprotin forming the base in mucous. It is found in
cartilage, connective tissue, saliva, salivary glands, and tendon.

MUCOPERIOSTEUM: Connective tissue having a mucous surface.

MUCOPERIOSTEUM MEMBRANE: The covering of bone, consisting of
periosteum with a mucous surface.

MUCOUS: The viscous secretion of the mucous glands. Covers the
membranes of many cavities and passages.

MUCOUS MEMBRANE: A layer of tissue lining cavities and passages,
containing fluid secreting cells.

MULTIPOLAR NEURON: A neuron having many dendrites and one axon.

MUSCLE: A type of tissue divided by its function into involuntary (cardiac, plain, smooth unstriated) and voluntary (skeletal, striated, strided). Muscle contraction produces movement. Muscle consists of a fleshy portion and attachments, with the head attached to a fixed structure, the origin, and the insertion into a movable structure. Involuntary muscle, which is not under conscious control, consists of spindly-shaped cells arranged parallel and grouped into bundles, layers, or sheets, without the cross striations of other kinds of muscle.

MUSCLE POTENTIAL: The action potential in a muscle generated by a impulse after crossing the synapse, between a muscle and a neuron.

MUSCULOTUBAL CANAL: The canal divided by a thin plate of bone into canals for the auditory tube and tensor tympanic muscle.

MYELENCEPHALON: In embryo development, the posterior portion of the rhombencephalon (hindbrain) from which the fourth ventricle and medulla oblongata develop.

MYELIN: A white substance, simular to fat, which forms a coverning or sheath around medullated neurons.

MYLOHYOID: Pertaining to the hyoid bone and molar teeth.

MYLOHYOID LINE-MANDIBLE BONE: Extending up and backward on each side of the mandible bone from the mental symphysis, for the origin of the mylohyoid muscle.

MYLOHYOID GROOVE: Located on the medial inner surface of the mandible bone, containing the mylohyoid artery and nerve.

MYLOHYOID MUSCLE: A extrinsic suprahyoid larynx elevator forming the floor of the mouth cavity. ORIGIN- Mandible bone mylohyoid line. DIRECTION- Medial and downward. INSERTION- Hyoid bone body and medial raphe. ACTION- Raise the hyoid bone. NERVE- Trigeminal (V cranial).

MYLOGYOID NERVE: A motor branch of the inferior alveolar nerve, a branch of the maxillary nerve, the third and largest branch of the trigeminal (V cranial) nerve. Directed to the digastricus and mylohyoideus muscles.

MYOELASTIC AERODYMANIC THEORY: Proposes that the true vocal folds are set into vibration by the air stream from the lungs. The frequency of vibration depends upon their length in relation to their mass and tension.

MYOFIBRILLA: A tiny fiber in muscle tissue, lying parallel to the cellular long axis from one cell to another. pl. myofibrillae.

MYOLOGY: The study of muscles.

MYONEURAL JUNCTION: (NEUROEFFECTOR JUNCTION) The point where a nerve fiber and muscle meet.

MYOTOME: (MYOTOMERE) In embryo development, the portion of a somite which develops into muscle.

MYRINGOSCOPE: (AURISCOPE) (OTOSCOPE) Instrument for visual examination of the external ear canal and tympanic membrane (eardrum).

N

Na: Symbol for sodium, a metallic element being soft, silver, white, and alkaline.

NAKED FIBERS: (GRAY FIBERS) (REMAK FIBERS) Robert Remak, German Neurologist. Unmyelinated nerve fibers in the gray matter portion of the brain and spinal cord, with the majority found in the autonomic nervous system.

NAPE: The back portion of the neck.

NARIS: One of the openings of the casal cavity. 2. A nostril. pl. nares.

NASAL: Pertaining to the nose.

NASAL ARCH: The arch formed by the nasal bones and the processes of the maxilla bone superior portion.

NASAL BONES: (BRIDGE OF THE NOSE) Two small oblong bones located side by side at point of midline and superior portion of the face. They articulate with the forntal bone and the ethmoid bone perpendicular plate.

NASAL CAPSULE: In embryo development, the cartilaginous capsules which enclose each of the sense organs. Such as the ears, eyes, and nasal cavities.

NASAL CARTILAGES: The cartilage forming the external portion of the nose. Consisting of the accessory nasal cartilages, greater and lesser alar; lateral nasal, nasal septal and vomeronasal cartilages.

NASAL CAVITY: Two narrow chambers divided by the nasal septum, being approximately symmetrical. They communicate externally by the nares (nostrils) and through the choanae, open into the nasopharynx behind. The septum anterior portion is cartilage and the posterior portion consists of the ethmoid bone perpendicular plate and the vomer bone. The floor of the cavity is concave, formed by the maxilla and palatine bones. The roof is pierced by the minute opening of the ethmoid bone cribriform plate, through which the olfactory nerves pass. The lateral walls of the cavity consist of the mucous membrane covered inferior, middle and superior conchae, and their passages containing minute openings through which they communicate with the paranasal sinuses. The labyrinthine surface of the conchae filter, moisens and warms the air as it is inhaled.

NASAL CONCHA: One of three scroll-like bones projecting medially from the lateral wall of the nasal cavity, each overlies a passage. The inferior concha is a face bone, the middle and superior conchae are processes of the ethmoid bone. pl. conchae.

NASAL CREST: The medial border of the maxilla bone which is thicker in front than behind. It forms a raised ridge which, along with the ridge from the opposite side, forms a groove holding the vomer bone.

NASAL EMINENCE: Located on the frontal bone vertical portion, above the nasal notch and between the supercillary ridges.

NASAL LAMINAE: In embryo development, the globular processes which fuse together and form the nasal septum.

NASAL MEATUS: The three passages formed by the nasal conchae.

NASAL NOTCH: Located at the medial limit on the maxilla bone anterior surface. The margin serves for the origin of the dilatator naris anterior muscle.

NASAL PITS: (OLFACTORY PIT) In embryo development, the pits formed by the growth of ectoderm areas under the forebrain. The pits divide into the lateral and medial nasal processes.

NASAL PLACODE: (OLFACTORY PLACODE) In embryo development, a

thickened plate of ectoderm which forms the first sign of the nasal organ.

NASAL PROCESS: (FRONTAL PROCESS-MAXILLA BONE) A plate which forms a portion of the lateral boundry of the nose. The medial surface forms a portion of the nasal cavity lateral wall.

NASAL SEPTAL: The partition between the openings of the nose. The bony portion is formed by the ethmoid and vomer bones and the cartilage portion formed by the medial crura of the greater alar cartilages and the sepal and vomeronasal cartilages.

NASAL SURFACE-LACRIMAL BONE: Contains a lengthwise furrow, the area in front of this forming a portion of the middle opening of the nose. The portion behind articulates with the ethmoid bone.

NASAL VESTIBULE: An area at the opening of the nose passages, lined withhair and sebaceous glands.

NASALIS MUSCLE: A muscle of the nose consisting of the alar and transverse portions. ORIGIN- Maxilla bone superior and lateral to the incisive fossa. DIRECTION- Medial and upward. INSERTION- Alar portion- ala of the nose. Transverse portion- aponeurosis of the procerus muscle. ACTION- Alar portion- widen nostril. Transverse portion- narrow nostrils. NERVE- Facial (VII cranial) buccal branch.

NASALITY: A voice disorder caused by faulty articulation due to inability to control the palate, insufficient palate closure caused by poor speaking habits, or insufficient palate tissue for proper isolation of the nasal and pharyngeal cavities.

NASOCILLIARY NERVE: A sensory branch of the ophthalmic nerve, the first division of the trigeminal (V cranial) nerve, which divides into the ethmoidal infrtrochlear, and long ciliary nerves, and the ciliary ganglion.

NASOLACINAL CANAL: A canal located between the inferior nasal conchae and lacrimal bone. Contains the nasolacrimal duct.

MASO-OPTIC FURROW: (NASO-OPTIC GROOVE) In embryo development, the furrow directed around the eyeball to the olfactory pit.

NASOPHARYNX: The upper portion of the pharyngeal cavity, bounded inferiorly at the level of the soft palate and superiorly by the pharyngeal protuberance of the occipital bone and rostrum of the sphenoid bone. It communicates with the auditory tube (Eustachian) and the conchae of the nasal cavities.

NASUS: See NOSE.

NATURAL LEVEL: (HABITUAL LEVEL) (PITCH LEVEL) The laryngeal tone that varies in pitch over a music range of two octaves. This level is located approximately one-fourth up the total singing range.

NERCK; The constricted portion of the body which connects the head with the body. 2. A narrow portion of any structure serving to join parts. 3. The area between the crown and root of a tooth.

NEOPALLIUM: (ISOCORTEX) The portion of the cerebral cortex which is non-olfactory, composed of six layers of cell and fiber tissue.

NERVE: A group of nerve fibers in a bundle or group. Each bundle is covered by a sheath of connective tissue throogh which stimuli are communicated from the central nervous system to the periphery, or the reverse.

NERVE CELL: A cell of the nervous system, either egg or pear shaped, giving off one process. 2. The cell body of a neuron.

NERVE CELL BODY: The nucleus, enclosed or surrounded by cytoplasm.

NERVE CENTER: A ganglionic or cerebrospinal system, beginning or controlling a function.

NERVE ENDING: The termination of a nerve, as an end process.

NERVE FIBER: The long process of a nerve cell.

NERVE PLEXUS: A group of nerves which are concentrated and intertwined.

NERVOUS SPINOSUS: (RAMUS MENINGEUS) A sensory branch of the mandibular nerve, the third and largest division of the trigeminal (V cranial) nerve. Directed to the dura mater and mastoid air cells.

NERVOUS SYSTEM: The complete nervous apparatus of the body consisting of the brain, spinal cord, ganglia and nerve fibers. Inc Includes the motor and sensory terminals which coordinate motor and sensory impulses.

NERVOUS TISSUE: Consists of groups of specialized cells in nerves

and nerve centers. They are capable of being irriated by modification of their chemical-electro composition.

NERVUS INTERMEDIUS: (GLOSSOPALATINE NERVE) A portion of the
facial (VII cranial) nerve between the facial nerve root and the
auditory (VIII cranial) nerve, containing both parasympathic and
sensory fibers.

NEURAL: Pertaining to nerves or nervous tissue.

NEURAL ARCH: (VERTEBRAL ARCH) The arch of a vertebra, formed by
the laminae and pedicles.

NEURAL CREST: (GANGLION RIDGE) In embryo development, a cellular band lateral to the neural tube for the origin of the spinal ganglia, and sympathic division of the autonomic nervous system.

NEURAL CURRENT: The electrical transmission along a nerve fiber
across a synapse.

NEURAL FOLD: (MEDULLARY FOLD) In embryo development, two folds,
one on each side of the neural plate. Through embryo development
in the third and fourth week, the folds join each other to form the
neural tube.

NEURAL GROOVE: In embryo development, the medial groove formed
by the thickened ectoderm as the neural folds are developed.

NEURAL PLATE: (MEDULLARY PLATE) In embryo development, a plate
of thickened ectoderm with the caudal portion forming the spinal
cord and the rostral end forming the brain; the origin of the central nervous system.

NEURAL TUBE: In embryo development, the tube formed by the fusion
of neural folds in the third and fourth week, forming the central
nervous system with the exception of the blood vessels and meninges.

NEURILEMMA: A thin myelin sheath coverning the peripheral nerves.

NEUROBLAST: In embryo development, a primitive embryo cell which
developes into a nerve cell.

NEUROCHRONXIC THEORY: (HUSSON'S THEORY) Proposes that each
vibratory cycle of the true vocal folds is initated by a nerve impulse
transmitted from the brain to the vocalis muscle by the vagus
(X cranial) nerve, recurrent branch.

NEUROCRANIUM: The portion of the complete skull enclosing the brain.

NEUROCYTE: A neuron or nerve cell.

NEUROEFFECTOR JUNCTION: (MYONEURAL JUNCTION) The point where a nerve fiber and muscle meet.

NEUROFIBRIL: A tiny fiber within a nerve cell.

NEUROFIBRILLA: The thread-like fibrils extending out in all directions in the cytoplasm of a nerve cell body. pl. neurofibrillae.

NEUROGLIA: Tissue of the central nervous system that is non-nerve, including the astrocytes, microglia, and oligodendrocytes.

NEUROGLIA CELLS: The mossy and spider cells. They form a web of tissue for support of nervous tissue.

NEUROLOGY: The study of the nervous system.

NEUROLYMPH: Cerebrospinal fluid.

NEUROMERE: In embryo development, a number of thickened portions on the rhombencephalon, matching the spinal cord segments and nerves.

NEUROMUSCULAR SPINDLE: A type of sensory nerve terminal between muscle fibers, usually near a muscle and tendon junction. The spindle responds to passive muscle length caused by tension.

NEURON: The basic structural unit of the nervous system. Consists of an axon, cell body, and dendrites. Classified as aggerent (sensory) directed to the brain or spinal cord or efferent (motor), directed away from the brain or spinal cord.

NEUTROCLUSION: In Angles classification system, Class I- A normal jaw relationship with abnormal teeth positions.

NIGRA: The gray matter between the dorsal and pedal portions of the crus cerebri.

NISSL BODIES: (NISSL GRANULES) Franz Nissal, Neurologist. Substance found by the staining of a nerve cell which forms the reticulum of a nerve cell cytoplasm.

NODE: A knob or protuberance. A point of constriction, or a small rounded organ.

NODE OF RAVNIER: A point along a nerve cell where the myelin sheath is broken and the nerve is exposed. The impulse jumps from node to node and thus increases speed.

MODOSE: To have nodes or projections.

NODOSE GANGLION: (INFERIOR GANGLION) An enlargement of the vagus (X cranial) nerve near the jugular foramen. From here motor and sensory fibers connect with the first and second cervical nerves, hypoglossal (XII cranial) nerve, and the sympathetic ganglion.

NODULE: A small node. 2. An aggregation of cells.

NODULUS: A small area of tissue. pl. noduli.

NOISE: Undesirable sound consisting of irregular frequencies with no periodicity and no definable fundamental frequency.

NOMENCLATURE: A system of naming organs, parts, or structures.

NORADRENALIN: See adrenal glands.

NOSE: (NASUS) A specialized organ of smell, and the entrance to the respiratory tract which filters, moisens and warms the air. The external portion is a pyramidal shaped bone and cartilage lined with mucous membrane. The two openings are separated by the nasal septum. Internally the septum divides the nose into two chambers. each chamber containing three passages. Opening into the middle passage are the anterior, ethmoid and maxillary sinuses. Opening into the superior passage are the posterior ethmoids, and sphenoids.

NOSE CARTILAGES: The framework of the nose. Consists of two greater alar, two lateral, and one lesser alar (sesamoid), septum and vomernasal cartilages.

NOSE MUSCLES: Consists of the depressor septi, dilatator naris anterior, dilator naris posterior, nasalis, procerus. They are helpful in facial expression but contribute little to speech production.

NOSTRIL: One of the external openings of the nose.

NOTCH: A deep indentation.

NOTCH OF RIVINUS: August Rivinus, Anatomist. A notch in the superior portion of the annular ring which holds the tympanic membrane (eardrum) at the edge of the external ear canal.

NOTOCHORD: In embryo development,. a column of cells developed from the mesoderm forming the primitive axial skeleton.

NOTOCHORD CANAL: In embryo development, a tunnel from the embryo head to the primitive pit.

NUCHA: The base, or nape of the neck.

NUCLEAR MEMBRANE: The outer layer of the nucleus.

NUCLEOLUS: A round shaped body in the nucleus of a cell.

NUCLEOPROTEIN: The combination of nucleic acid and one of the body proteins.

NUCLEUS: A spherical body located in the center of the cell. It is surrounded by a nuclear envelope or membrane, and contains pores that allow communication with the cytoplasm.

NUCLEUS AMBIGOUS: A group of nerve cells in the medulla oblongta. They form the motor nucleus of the glossopharyngeal (IX cranial), vagus (X cranial), and accessory (XI cranial) nerves directed to the larynx and pharynx.

NUCLEUS FASTIGII: A mass of gray matter over the roof of the fourth ventricle which receives fibers from the auditory nerve vestibular branch, (VIII cranial).

NUEL'S SPACE: (SPACE OF NUEL) Jean P. Nuel, Belgian Otologist. The space between the outer pillar and outer phalangeal cells. It provide a passage for nerve fibers and endolymph fluid, which baths and nourishes the inner cells of the organ of Corti.

O

OBLIQUE: A direction, diagonal or slanting.

OBLIQUE LINE-MANDIBLE BONE: A faint ridge running upward from each mental tubercle on the body.

OBLIQUE LINE- LARYNX: A slight line which runs down and forward on the thyroid cartilage. This serves for attachemtn of extrinsic laryngeal muscles.

OBLIQUE LINE-THYROID CARTILAGE: The line on the external surface of each lamina of the thyroid cartilage. This is the area for
attachment of muscles.

OBLIQUE AURICULAE MUSCLE: ORIGIN- Concha of the external ear.
INSERTION- Above the concha at the cranial surface. NERVE-
Facial (VII cranial) posterior auricular branch.

OBTURATOR FORAMEN: (THYROID FORAMEN) The opening between
the ischium and pubis bones.

OCCIPITAL: Pertaining to the back of the head.

OCCIPITAL BONE: A single trapezoid-shaped bone located at, and
forming the inferior and posterior portion of the cranium. In the
inferior portion is a large opening   the magnum foramen through
which the accessory nerves, medulla oblongata, membranes, and
vertebral arteries pass. Its major portions are the basilar, lateral,
and squama. It articulates with the parietal, spenoid, and temporal
bones and the first cervical vertebra (atlas).

OCCIPITAL CONDYLE: The round-like process on each side of the
occipital bone near the foramen magnum which articulates with
the first cervical vertebra (atlas).

OCCIPITAL LOBE -CEREBRUM: The lobe located at the posterior of
the cerebrum, from the posterior pole to the parieto-occipital
fissure.

OCCIPITAL MAGNUM: (FORAMEN MAGNUM) The large oval opening
in the occipital bone connecting the cranial cavity with the vertebral canal.

OCCLUDE: To close tightly, or join together.

OCCLUSION: State of being closed. 2. Relationship of the teeth with
the mandible and maxillary bones in normal closure.

OCTAVE: Interval between two frequencies, one being twice as large
as the other.

OCULAR: Pertaining to the eyes or eyesight.

OCULOMOTOR NERVE: (OCILOMOTORIUS NERVE) III cranial, a motor
nerve with its origin from the nucleus in the floor of the cerebral
aqueduct. Supplying motor fibers to four of the extrinsic muscles

of the eyeball, with parasympathetic fibers supplying two intrinsic muscles of the eye.

OCULOMOTOR NUCLEUS: A group of nerve cells in the superior colliculus from which the oculomotor (III cranial) nerve arises.

ODENTOSIS: The development or the eruption of the teeth.

ODONTOBLAST: A cell forming the outer layer of the dental papilla.

ODONTOID PROCESS: A toothlike projection from the superior surface of the body of the second cervical vertebra.

Ohm: George Ohm. Unit of resistance of a conductor in which one volt produces a current flow of one ampere. Also used to denote resistance to the transference of other forms of energy. Example- mechanical, acoustical resistance has a magnitude of one acoustical ohm when a sound pressure of one microbar produces a volume velocity of one cubic centimeter per second.

OHTHALMOSCOPE MIRROR: An instrument used for the examination of the interior of the eye.

OLFACTION: The sense of smell. 2. The act of smelling.

OLFACTORY BULB: The expanded anterior olfactory tract which rests on the ethmoid bone cribriform plate.

OLFACTORY FORAMEN: The opening in the ethmoid bone cribriform plate for passage of the olfactory nerves.

OLFACTORY NERVE: (OLFACTORII NERVE) I cranial, a sensory nerve arising as a short bundle of fibers from the deep processes of the olfactory cells of mucous membrane. They collect into approximately twenty branches that pierce the ethmoid bone cribriform plate in two groups and form synapses with cells of the olfactory bulb.

OLFACTORY PIT: (NASAL PITS) In embryo development, the pits formed by the growth of ectoderm areas under the forebrain. The pits devide into the lateral and medial nasal processes.

OLFACTORY PLACODE: (NASAL PLACODE) In embryo development, a thickened plate of ectoderm which forms the first sign of the nasal organ.

OLFACTORY TRACT: A band of fibers directed from the olfactory bulb to the frontal lobe inferior surface.

OLIGODENDROCYTE: (OLIGODENDROGLIA) Neuroglial cells with a few processes forming a portion of the central nervous system. May assist in the formation of myelin sheaths.

OLIVARY: Shaped like an olive.

OLIVARY BODY: A rolled sheet of gray matter enclosing white matter. 2. A round-shaped mass in the interlateral portion of the medulla oblongata.

OLIVARY NUCLEUS: A group of nerve cells in the olive complex of the medulla.

OLIVO-COCHLEA BUNDLE: (BUNDLE OF RASMUSSEN) G. L. Rasmussen) A bundle of efferent nerve fibers between the cochlea and the olivary complex.

OLIVOSPINAL TRACT: An ascending tract of the spinal cord. Originats near the inferior olivary nucleus in the medulla oblongata and sends motor proprioceptive impulses of reflex activities.

OMOHYOID MUSCLE: A extrinsic infrahyoid larynx elevator. ORIGIN- Scapula bone upper margin. DIRECTION- Forward and horizontal. INSERTION- Hyoid bone, lower border of the greater cornu. ACTION- Depresses hyoid bone. NERVE- Hypoglossal (XII cranial).

ONTOGENY: Complete developmental history of an individual organism.

OOGENESIS: The origin and formation of the ovum.

OPERCULUM: A covering, or lid of the insula. 2. Convolutions of the cerebrum with the margins separated by the lateral cerebral (Sylvian) fissure. pl. opercula.

OPHTHALMIC NERVE: A sensory nerve, the first of three divisions of the trigeminal (V cranial) nerve, which divides into the frontal, lacrimal and nasociliary branches. Supplies the cornea, eyelid, iris, lacrimal gland, paranasal sinuses, and skin of the superior facial area with sensation of pain and touch.

OPTIC CHIASMA: The X-shaped crossing of the optic nerve fibers. Located at the anterior wall and floor of the third ventricle.

OPTIC FORAMEN: The opening in the sphenoid bone small wing for passage of the ophthalmic artery and optic (II cranial) nerve.

OPTIC NERVE: (OPICUS NERVE) II cranial, a sensory nerve with origin in the optic chiasma. Distribution of the fibers is from the medial half of each retina and are direct, or uncrossed. They continue to central connections and fourth order neurons, terminating in the occipital cortex.

OPTIC TRACT: A band of fibers forming the middle extension of the optic (II cranial) nerve, extending to the thalamus geniculate body.

ORAL GROOVE: (STOMODEUM) In embryo development, the infolding of the ectoderm which forms the primitive mouth.

ORAL PLATE: (BUCCOPHARYNGEAL MEMBRANE) In embryo development, it forms the separation between the foregut and oral groove, the location for the opening into the mouth.

ORAL VESTIBULE: The area externally between the cheeks and lips, and internally between the gums and teeth.

ORAL CAVITY PROPER: Bounded anterioraly, and laterally by the teeth and alveolar processes, inferiorly by the floor, formed by the tongue, posteriorly by the isthmus of faucium, and superiorly by the hard and soft palates.

ORBICULAR: Pertaining to the circular muscles of the mouth.

ORBICULARIS ORIS MUSCLE: A ring of muscle of the mouth for facial expression. ORIGIN- Mandible bone canine fossa and nasal septum. DIRECTION- All directions around the mouth. INSERTION- Buccinator and muscles surrounding the mouth. ACTION- Closes the lips. NERVE- Facial (VII cranial).

ORBIT: The bony cavity containing the eye organ.

ORBITAL-FRONTAL BONE: (HORIZONTAL PART) The portion of the frontal bone composed of the two orbital plates. These are separated by the ethmoid notch which receives the cribriform plate of the ethmoid bone. The plates form the vaults of the orbital cavity.

ORBITAL BRANCHES: Sensory branches of the pterygopalatine nerves, a branch of the maxillary nerve, the second division of the trigeminal (V cranial) nerve. It is directed to the ethmoid sinus, eye orbit periosteum, and sphenoid sinus.

ORBITAL NERVE: (ZYGOMATIC NERVE) A sensory branch of the sec second division of the trigeminal (V cranial) nerve, which divides into the zygomaticofacial and zygomaticotemporal branches. They supply the skin of the cheek and skin at the side of the forehead.

ORBITAL PROCESS-PALATINE BONE: Located on the superior portion of the palatine bone, being pyramid-shaped with one surface forming a portion of the orbit floor.

ORBITAL SURFACE-MAXILLA BONE: (SUPERIOR SURFACE) A smooth and triangle-shaped area forming most of the orbital (superior) cavity floor, with the medial border articulating with the ethmoid, lacrimal, and palatine bones.

ORBITAL PROCESS-ZYGOMATIC BONE: A strong thick plate forming the orbital surface of the maxilla bone and the great wing of the sphenoid bone forms a portion of the floor and lateral wall of the orbit.

ORDINATE: The vertical line, or vertical axis on a graph showing the relationship of two values, such as date and time.

ORGAN: A part of the body that performs a specific function.

ORGAN OF CORTI: (SPIRAL ORGAN OF CORTI) Alfonso Corti, Italian Anatomist. The recepter, sensory, transmitter system of the ear, located in the cochlea and resting of the basilar membrane. It consists of hair cells and rod-shaped cells which extend into the endolymph fluid of the scala media (cochlea duct). Projecting over the cells from the spiral lamina is a roof-like coverning, the tectorial membrane. Attached to the membrane are the hairs of the cell so that through vibration of the basilar membrane the hair cells relax and stretch. The auditory nerve (VIII cranial) cochlea nerve branch contains fibers arising in the spiral ganglion nerve cells from the modiolus. These are directed to the brain, some end in the organ hair cells, and others around the hair cells of the organ of Corti.

ORGAN SYSTEM: A complete system consisting of at least two organs combining to exhibit functional unity.

ORGANIC: Pertaining to an organ or number of organs,

ORIFICE: The entrance or exit of a body cavity.

ORIGIN- The plate of attachment of a muscle, which remains relatively fixed during contraction.

OROPHARYNX: The middle portion of the pharyngeal cavity, bounded by the soft palate and the level of the hyoid bone. It communicates with the oral cavities by the fauces. Its lateral wall, between the two palatine arches is the palatine tonsil.

OS: A mouth or opening. 2. Used with an adjective to designate a specific type bone, or bone structure.

OS COXAE: (HIP BONE) (INNOMINATUM) Consists of three major portions; ilium, ischium, and pubis. pl. ilia, ischia, pubes.

OS PUBIS: (PUBIC BONE) The anterior portion of the os coxae (hip bone) on each side, which articulate at midline with the symphysis.

OSSEOUS: Being of bone. 2. Bony.

OSSEOUS LABYRINTH: (BONY LABYRINTH) The cavities of the internal ear in the temporal bone petrous portion. Lined with periosteum and containing perilymph fluid. It consist of the cochlea, semicircular canals, and vestibule.

OSSEOUS SPIRAL LAMINA: (SPIRAL LAMINA) A bony ledge or shelf consisting of two very thin plates of bone between which canals for transmission of the auditory nerve fibers are located. It projects from the modiolus into the cochlea canal, dividing it into the lower portion the scala tympani, and the upper portion the scala vestibule. It is narrow at the apex end, wide toward the basal end.

OSSICLE: A small bone,

OSSICULAR CHAIN: The three tiny bones of the tympanic cavity (middle ear); the incus (anvil), malleus (hammer) and stapes (stippup). They transmit sound vibrations to the inner ear fluid and protect the inner ear from excessive vibrations.

OSSIFIC: Becoming, or forming bone.

OSSIFICATION: Formation of bone. The changing of fibrous tissue into bone.

OSSIFICATION CENTER: The place where bone ossification begins.

OSSEOUS PORTION-AUDITORY TUBE: Begins in the carotid wall of the tympanic cavity (middle ear) and gradually narrows, ending at the junction of the squama and petrous portions of the temporal bone as a jagged margin. This serves for the attachment of the cartilaginous portion.

OSTEOSEPTUM: The bony portion of the nasal septum.

OSTEOBLAST: Cell which arises, and as it grows is associated with the making of bone.

OSTEOLOGY: The study of bone.

OSTIUM: A door or opening in a tubular organ. 2. Opening into two body cavities.

OTOCONIUM: (OTOLITHS) (EAR DUST) Minute dust-like particles of calcium carbonate in one layer in the maculae of the inner ear. As head position changes the particles roll against hair cells to send nerve impulses to the brain as to body orientation and equilibrium.

OTOSCOPE: (AURISCOPE) (MYRINGOSCOPE) Instrument for visual examination of the external ear canal and tympanic membrane (eardrum).

OUT OF PHASE: Produced when two tones of the same frequency and intensity are presented with the period of compression and rarefaction of each separated by half a cycle (90^0). With the tone 180^0 out of phase they will cancel each other out with an amplitude of zero.

OUTER HAIR CELLS: Hair cells which rest on the outer edge of the basilar membrane in the organ of Corti.

OVAL WINDOW: (FENESTRA VESTIBULI) A oval shaped opening in the labyrinthic wall above the fenestra rotunda (round window) opening into the vestibule of the inner ear.

OVARIES/TESTES: Glands of the endocrine system, The testes produce testosterone, important in development of male secondary sexual characteristics. The ovaries produce estrogen, important for development of female secondary sexual characteristics and progesterone, which initiates and menstrual cycle.

OVERTONE: Complex tones, produced by such generators as vibrating strings, contain component frequencies that are integral multiples of the lowest frequency. The first component is the fundamental frequency, or first harmonic and the others are overtones.

OVERBITE: When the jaws are in centric occlusion, the vertical extension of the upper teeth is over the lower teeth.

OVUM: The reproductive cell of the female which may be fertilized.

OXIDIZE: To combine chemically with oxygen.

P

PACINIAN CORPUSLES: Filippo Pacini, Italian Anatomist. A seosory organ of connective tissue around a nerve ending, found in joints and tendons, functioning as receptors of pressure.

PAD OF BICHAT: (BUCCAL FAT PAD) (SUCTORIAL PAD) Farie F. Bichat, French Anatomist. A deposit of fat in the cheeks superficial to the buccinator muscle. This pad is prominent in infants and assists in the sucking action.

PALATAL: A consonant classification of articulators used, and the position they are in.

PALATAL RAPHE: Slight ridges on the hard palate on the posterior portion of the alveolar arch.

PALATAL VAULT; The arch-like dome formed by the hard palate, being thick at its anterior and lateral margins, thining toward midline forming a dome. The height determins the acoustics of the oral cavity and are classified by shape as ovoid, trapezoid and triangular.

PALATE: (ROOF OF THE MOUTH) A bony plate separating the nasal and oral cavities. It consists of the hard palate in front and the soft palate behind. Its function is to change the degree of coupling between the nasopharynx and vocal tract.

PALATE PLATE: The portion of the palatine bone forming the lateral half of the roof of the mouth.

PALATINE ARCHES: The arch-shaped folds of mucous membrane, the glossopalatine, and pharyngopalatine arches, forming the lateral margins of the faucial pharyngeal isthmuses.

PALATE BONE: (PALATINE BONE) Two irregular somewhat L-shaped bones forming a portion of the lateral wall and floor of the nasal cavity, the floor of the orbital cavity and the posterior portion of the hard palate. The horizontal portion is quadrilateral-shaped having two surfaces, the inferior concave surface forms a portion of the hard palate and the concave superior surface forms a portion of the nasal cavity floor. It articulates with the ethmoid, inferior nasal concha, maxilla, sphenoid, and vomer bones.

PALATINE GROOVE: Located on the inner surface of the maxilla bone palatine process containing the palatine nerve.

PALATINE NERVE: (GREATER PALATINE NERVE) A sensory branch of the pterygopalatine nerve which is a branch of the maxillary nerve, the second division of the trigeminal (V cranial) nerve. From the pterygopaline ganglion it is directed to the gums and the mucous membrane of the hard and soft palate.

PALATINE PROCESS-MAXILLA BONE: A strong, thick, horizontal process projecting medial from the nasal surface of the bone. It joints at the midline with its opposite side forming approximately three quarters of the ranal cavity floor and roof of the mouth, being thicker in front than behind.

PALATINE RAPHE: (MEDIAL RAPHE) A faint line, or ridge in the midline of the palate.

PALATINE TONSIL: An almond-shaped mass of lymphoid tissue on each side of the oral cavity between the palatoglossal and palatopharyngeal arches. They are covered by mucous membrane and contain minute, tube-like depressions and lymph follicles acting to filter and destroy bacteria entering the mouth.

PALATOGLOSSAL ARCH:(GLOSSOPALATINE ARCH)(ANTERIOR PILLAR OF FAUCES) The anterior one of two folds of mucous membrane. It is formed by the downward curve from the soft palate to the side of the tongue base, enclosing the palatoglossal muscle.

PALATOGLOSSUS MUSCLE: (GLOSSOPALATINE MUSCLE) A muscle of the soft palate. ORIGIN- Soft palate anterior surface. DIRECTION- Downward, forward and lateral. INSERTION- Side of the tongue. ACTION- Raises tongue, constricts the fauces. NERVE- Vagus (X cranial) pharyngeal plexus.

PALATOPHARYNGEAL ARCH: (POSTERIOR PILLAR OF FAUCES) The posterior one of the two folds of mucous membrane, This is formed by the downward curve from the soft palate to the side of the tongue.

It encloses the palatopharyngeal muscle.

PALATOPHARYNGEUS: (PHARYNGOPALATINUS MUSCLE) A long bundle of muscle fibers forming the pharyngopalatine arch of the soft palate. ORIGIN- Soft palate. DIRECTION- Lateral, downward. INSERTION- Dorsal border of thyroid cartilage and aponeurosis. ACTION- Depresses the palate, elevates the larynx. NERVE- Vagus (X cranial), pharyngeal plexus.

PALATUM DURUM: (HARD PALATE) The anterior ridge portion of the palate formed by the medial projection of the maxilla bone palatine processes. Meeting at midline it forms approximately three quarters of the bony roof of the mouth, which forms the floor of the nasal cavity. It is covered by mucous membrane and rugae (small ridges or wrinkles).

PALLIUM: Gray matter that covers the cerebral hemispheres.

PALPATION: The application of light pressure with the fingers to the external surface of the body.

PANCREAS: A ductless gland of the endocrine system. Located behind the stomach in front of the first and second lumbar vertebrae. It is hammer shaped, consisting of the head, body, and tail. Secretions consist of pancreatic fluid to aid intestinal digestion, in addition to a small group of cells, the Islets of Langerhans, which secrete glucagon and insulin that is absorbed by the blood stream to regulate the retention and storage of sugar.

PAPILLA: A nipple-shaped, small elevation or projection found on the tongue. Consists of three types; filiform, fungiform and vallate. pl. papillae.

PARACENTRAL LOBULE: The posterior portion of the superior frontal gyrus directed into the parietal lobe.

PARALLEL MUSCLE: Bundles of muscle fibers that are parallel to the long axis of the muscle and terminate at a flat tendon. They have a great range of motion and may shorten up to one half their length.

PARANASAL SINUSES: (ACCESSORY SINUSES) The ethmoidal, frontal, maxillary, and sphenoidal sinuses of the nose lined by ciliated mucous membrane.

PARASAGITTAL: Being longitudinal, or paralled to the sagittal plane.

PARASYMPATHETIC DIVISION-AUTONOMIC NERVOUS SYSTEM: (CRANIOSACRAL DIVISION-AUTONOMIC NERVOUS SYSTEM) This division is connected to the central nervous system by efferent fibers from the facial (VII cranial), glossopharyngeal (IX cranial), vagus (X cranial) nerves and fibers from the second, third and fourth sacral segment of the sinal cord and are usually located peripherially near the structures they serve. This system tends to act to restore reserves by slowing the heart beat and the alimentary tract and glands become more active and is the innervator of involuntary muscle, directed to the eye muscles, glands of the gums, lips, salivary glands and soft palate.

PARATHYROID GLANDS: Ductless glands of the endocrine system, located as two pair of oval-shaped masses of cells. The inferior pair, behind the lower pole of the thyroid gland, with the superior pair at the level of the cricoid cartilage at the union of the esophagus and pharynx. The gland secretes parathormone, a hormone rich in protein which regulates calcium and phosphorus levels in the blood.

PARAXIAL: Along the side of an axis.

PARAXIAL MESODERM: In embryo development, the mesoderm located along the neural tube and notochord.

PARENCHYMA: The essential part of an organ that shows its function.

PARIETAL: The walls of cavities or organs. 2. Forming or situated on a wall. 3. The parietal bones of the cranium, or the lobes of the brain near these bones.

PARIETAL BONES; The two bones forming the backroof and sides of the cranium, The external surface is convex, with the internal surface concave containing depressions which match the cerebral convolutions. The bone articulates with five bones, the frontal, occipital, opposite parietal, sphenoid, and temporal bones.

PARIETAL EMINENCE: The convexity on the exterior surface of the parietal bone.

PARIETAL LOBE-CEREBRUM: The upper central lobe of the cerebral cortex, bounded behind by the parieto-occipital fissure.

PARIETAL PLEURA: (COSTAL PLEURA) Serous membrane lining the walls of the thoracic cavity.

PARIETO-OCCIPITAL FISSURE: A fissure between the occipital and parietal lobes of the cerebrum.

PARIETO-OCCIPITAL SULCUS: Located in each hemisphere. Directed upward from the calcarine sulcus, between the occipital and parietal lobes.

PAROTIC DUCT: (STENSEN'S DUCT) Niels Stensen, Danish Physican. Originates at the parotic gland, crosses the masseter muscle, passes through the buccenator muscle, and opens on the internal surface of the cheek opposite the upper second molar tooth. The duct is for secretion of saliva in the mouth.

PAROTID GLAND: The largest of the three salivary glands of the mouth. Located below and in front of the external ear enclosed on a sheath, the parotid fascia.

PAROTID NERVE BRANCHES: Sensory branches of the auriculotemporal nerve, a branch of the mandibular nerve, the third and largest division of the trigeminal (V cranial) nerve, directed to the parotid gland.

PARS: Designation of a larger area of a organ or structure. 2. A part. pl. partes.

PARS BASILARIS: (OCCIPITAL BONE BASILAR PORTION) A quadrilateral portion of the bone projecting forward and upward from the magnum forament, articulating with the sphenoid bone.

PARS EXTERNA: The outer portion of the external auditory canal directed inward, forward, and upward.

PARS FLACCIDA: (SHRAPNELL'S MEMBRANE) Henry J. Shrapnell, English Anatomist. The superior triangular portion of the tympanic membrane (eardrum), between the malleolar folds, filling the notch of Rivinus.

PARS INTERNA: The medial portion of the external auditory canal directed inward, forward, and downward.

PARS LATERALIS: (OCCIPITAL BONE-LATERAL PARTS: Located at the sides of the magum foramen. The condyles are on the under surface for articulation with the superior facets of the first cervical vertebra (atlas).

PARS MEDIA: The middle portion of the external auditory canal, directed inward and backward.

PARS OBLIQUE: The lower fibers of the cricothyroid muscle. These are directed upward and back to insert into the anterior margin of the inferior cornu of the thyroid cartilage.

PARS RECTA: The upper fibers of the cricothyroid muscle. These are directed vertical upward, inserting along the lower margin of the thyroid lamina.

PARS TENSA: The largest portion of the tympanic membrane (eardrum). This portion is tightly streched in contrast with the triangular flaccid part above it.

PARTIAL: In acoustics, a component of a complex tone.

PASSAGE: A channel or meatus.

PASSAVANT'S BAR: (PAD) Philip G. Passavant, German Surgeon. A bulge of muscle formed by fibers from the palatopharyngeal and superior constrictor. It is present on the posterior wall of the pharynx when these muscles are contracted.

PATENT: Apparent or evident. 2. Open, not closed.

PATHOLOGY: A biological science dealing with the nature of disease, its courses and its effects.

PECTINATE: Shaped like a comb.

PECTINATA HABENULA: (PEFORATE HABENULA) The outer most portion of the basilar membrane of the organ of Corti.

PECTINIFORM: Having teeth like a comb.

PECTORAL: Pertaining to the chest. The muscles that form the chest.

PECTORAL GIRDLE: The clavicle and scapula bones.

PECTORALIS MAJOR MUSCLE: A fanshaped thorax and of inhalation. ORIGIN- Clavical and sternum bones, ribs one through six. DIRECTION- Upward and lateral. INSERTION-Humerus bone head. ACTION-Raise ribs. NERVE-Lower cervical and first thoracic.

PECTORALIS MINOR MUSCLE: A fanshaped muscle of the thorax and of inhalation. ORIGIN- Ribs two through five. DIRECTION- Upward. INSERTION-Scapula bone coracoid process. ACTION- Raise ribs. NERVE- Cervical seven and eight.

PEDICLE: Bony process, projecting backward from the body of a vertebra, connecting with lamina on each side forming the root of the arch. 2. A process, or projection that resembles a foot or stalk.

PEDUNCLE: (PEDUNCLUS) Collections of nerve fibers running between different areas in the nervous system. 2. Stem-like.

PEFORATE HABENULA: (PECTINATA HABENULA) The outer most portion of the basilar membrane on which the organ of Corti rest.

PELVIS: The structure formed by the os coxae (hip bones), coccyx, sacrum, and their ligaments. Serves as a support for the vertebral column and articulation with the lower limbs. 2. A basin shaped cavity or structure.

PELVIC: Pertaining to the pelvis. pl. pelves.

PELVIC GIRDLE: The bony structure formed by the os coxae (hip bones) which articulate together at the pubic sumphysis.

PENNATE: Penniform, or feather shaped.

PENNIFORM: Feather-like.

PENNIFORM MUSCLE: Bundles of muscle fibers converging on a tendon in a feather-shape. Power is combined from all the contracting fibers, and the length is equal to the amount of contraction.

PERICARDIAL CAVITY: The space located in the abdomen between the parietal and visceral portions of the serous pericardium.

PERICARDIUM: A fibroserous, membranous double sac enclosing the heart and the origin of the great blood vessels. Composed of an inner serous layer and outer fibrous layer. The inner space is the pericardinal cavity, filled with serous fluid. The base is attached to the diaphragm, and the apex extends upward to the first division of the great blood vessels. In front it attaches to the sternum bone, lateral to the mediastinal pleura, and posteriorly to the esophagus, main bronchi and trachea.

PERICHONDRIUM: A membrane layer of fibrous tissue which covers the cartilage surface.

PERIKARYON: The cell body set off from the nucleus and processes.

PERILYMPH: A clearm thin, watery fluid; a portion of the cerebro-spinal fluid. This fills the scala tympani, scala vestibuli, and the semicircular canals.

PERIMYSIUM: A sheath of connective tissue around each primary bundle of skeletal muscle fibers.

PERIOD: The time required for an oscillating body to make one com-plete oscillating or vibratory cycle.

PERIODONTAL: Surrounding a tooth, especially its root.

PERIODONTIUM: The tissues in, and supporting the teeth, including alveolar bone, cementum, and gingiva (gums).

PERIOSTIUM: (FIBROUS MEMBRANE) The connective tissue coverning bones, except at articulating surfaces. The external layer contains numerous blood vessels, and the internal layer larger connective tissue cells. It serves as a support structure for blood vessels and attachment of ligaments, muscles and tendons.

PERIOTIC BONE: The mastoid and petrous portion of the temporal bone.

PERIPHERAL: The outside, or near the body surface.

PERIPHERAL NERVOUS SYSTEM: A portion of the nervous system. Consists of the twelve cranial nerves, and the thirty-one pair of spinal nerves including their roots and branches. They serve as connectors of "centers" by directing impulses away from, or toward the brain and spinal cord of the central nervous system.

PERIPHERY: Away from the center. The outer surface of the body.

PERISTALTIC ACTION: An involuntary, progressive squeezing move-ment.

PERISTALSIS: Successive waves of involuntary contraction passing along the walls of hollow muscular structures , forcing the contents onward.

PERITONEUM: The membranous lining of the abdominal cavity.

PERMANENT TEETH: (SECONDARY TEETH) The second set of teeth which appear from approximately the sixth through the twenty-fifth year. The thirty-two teeth include two canine, four incisor, six molar and four premolar in each jaw represented by the following dental formula:

157

I $\frac{2\text{-}2}{2\text{-}2}$	C $\frac{1\text{-}1}{1\text{-}1}$	PM $\frac{2\text{-}2}{2\text{-}2}$	M $\frac{3\text{-}3}{3\text{-}3}$

Approximate Eruption in Years

First molars	6-7	Second premolars	9-10
Central incisors	7-8	Canines	12-14
Lateral incisors	7-8	Second molars	12-15
First premolars	9-10	Third molars	17-25

PERPENDICULAR PLATE-ETHMOID BONE: (VERTICAL PLATE) A flat, thin polygonal-shaped plate descending from the under surface of the cribriform plate of the ethmoid bone forming a portion of the basal septum and deflected to one side slightly. The anterior border articulates with the crest of the nasal bones and spine of the frontal bone. The inferior border serves for the attachment of the septal cartilage of the nose.

PETROUS: Being hard, like a rock or stone.

PETROUS GANGLION: (INFERIOR GANGLION) (NODOSE GANGLION) Located in a depression in the temporal bone lower border. The ganglion contain cell bodies for sensory fibers of the glossopharyngeal (IX cranial) nerve.

PETROUS PORTION- TEMPORAL BONE: The hardest bone of the body located between the occipital and sphenoid bones. The interior portion contains the organs of hearing and equilibrium.

PHALANX: One of a set of plates formed by phalangeal cells, both inner and outer, forming the supporting structure of the hair cells in the organ of Corti. pl. phalanges.

PHARYNGEAL APONEUROSIS: The sheet of fibrous membrane in the pharynx wall. It is lined with mucous membrane and attached to the auditory (Eustachian) tube cartilage, medial pterygoid plate, temporal bone petrous portion, and the occipital bone tubercle.

PHARYNGEAL BRANCH: A sensory branch of the pterygopalatine nerves, a branch of the maxillary nerve, the second division of the trigeminal (V cranial) nerve. Directed to the nasal portion of the pharynx.

PHARYNGEAL BURSA: A small, blind sac on the lower portion of the pharyngeal tonsil.

PHARYNGEAL CANAL (PTERYGOID CANAL) Serves for transmission of the pterygoid nerves and vessels. It runs forward through the base of the sphenoid bone medial pterygoid plate, opening inferior and medial to the foramen rotundum.

PHARYNGEAL CAVITY: (PHARYNX) A musculomembranous tube extending from the base of the skull to the level of the sixth cervical vertebra behind, and in front to the cricoid cartilage. It is divided into the nasopharynx, the portion above the soft palate communicating with the posterior nares and auditory (Eustachian) tube; the middle portion, the oropharynx between the soft palate and upper edge of the epiglottis; and the laryngopharynx, being below the upper edge of the epiglottis and opening into the esophagus and larynx.

PHALANGEAL LEVATOR MUSCLES: Consists of the salpingopharyngeal and stylopharyngeal muscles.

PHARYNGEAL LUMEN: See Lumen.

PHARYNGEAL MUSCLES: Consists of the cricopharyngeal, inferior, middle, and superior constrictors, and the velopharyngeal muscles.

PHARYNGEAL NERVE BRANCHES: Sensory branches of the glossopharyngeal (IX cranial) nerve, directed to the pharynx and muscles.

PHARYNGEAL OSTIUM: (PHARYNGEUM TUBAEAUDITIUAE) The opening of the auditory tube, pharyngeal end.

PHARYNGEAL PLEXUS: A concentration of nerve fibers from the glossopharyngeal (IX cranial) and vagus (X cranial) nerves. Directed to the muscles of the pharynx and soft palate.

PHALANGEAL PROCESSES: Formed by the outward continuation of the flat plate-like heads of the outer rods which, along with the phalangeal processes of the Deiter's cells, form the delicate net-like reticular membrane in the organ of Corti.

PHARYNGEAL POUCHES: (BRANCHIAL ARCHES) (VISCERAL ARCHES) In embryo development, five pair of arches from which face and neck structures are formed. The mandibular, or first arch, forms the anterior portion of the tongue, lower lip, mandible bone and muscles of mastication. The hyoid or second arch, forms the hyoid bone lesser cornu, stapes bone, styoid process and stylohyoid ligament. The third arch forms the hyoid bone, greater cornu and the post-

erior portion of the tongue, The fourth arch forms the thyroid cartilage and from the fifth arch the arytenoid and cricoid cartilages is
formed.

PHARYNGEAL RAPHE: A band of connective tissue directed downward
from the skull for the attachment of constrictor muscle of the
pharynx.

PHARYNGEAL RECESS: (FOSSA OF ROSENMULLER) Johann C. Rosemuller, German Physician. A deep depression in the pharynx wall,
above and behind the auditory (Eustachian) tube.

PHARYNGEAL TONSIL: (ADENOIDS) A mass of lymphoid tissue in the
posterior wall of the pharynx.

PHARYNGEUM TUBAEAUDITIUAE: (PHARYNGEAL OSTIUM) The opening of the auditory tube pharyngeal end.

PHARYNGOPALATINUS MUSCLE: (PALATOPHARYNGEUS) A long bun-
dle of muscle fibers forming the pharyngopalatine arch of the soft
palate. ORIGIN- Soft palate. DIRECTION- Lateral, downward. IN-
SERTION- Dorsal border of the thyroid cartilage and aponeurosis.
ACTION- Depresses the palate, elecates the larynx. NERVE- Vagus
(X cranial), pharyngeal plexus.

PHARYNX: (PHARYNGEAL CAVITY) A musculomembranous tube extending from the base of the skull to the level of the sixth cervical
vertebra behind, and in front to the cricoid cartilage. It is divided
into the nasopharynx, the portion above the soft palate communicating with the posterior nares and auditory (Eustachian) tube: the
middle portion, the oropharynx between the soft palate and upper
edge of the epiglottis; and the laryngopharynx, being below the upper
edge of the epiglottis and opening into the esophagus and larynx.

PHASE: A measurement of vibratory motion. The relationship in time
between two or more sound waves. It is expressed as degrees of a
circle, a complete vibrating cycle being 360^0.

PHEOBASE: The minimum amount of electricity to produce stimulation.

PHILTRUM: The vertical groove at midline in the upper lip.

PHONATION: The production of sounds by the vibration of the true
vocal folds.

PHONE: An individual speech sound.

PHONEME: The smallest distinctive group or class of phones in a language.

PHONEMIC: The discrimination of distincitive speech sound in a language.

PHOTOCELL: An electronic device that is sensitive to light.

PHOTOMICROGRAPH: A photograph of a microscopic object, usually made with the aid of a microscope.

PHRENIC: Pertaining to the diaphragm.

PHRENIC NERVE: A motor and sensory nerve originating from the cervical plexus, directed to the diaphragm.

PHYLUM: One of the main divisions of the animal or plant kingdom.

PHYSIOLOGY: The study of the function of cells, organs, and tissues of a living organism.

PIA MATER: The inner, and most vascular portion of the three membranous layers coverning the brain and spinal cord. The space between the pia mater and the arachnoid (middle) layer contains cerebrospinal fluid.

PILLAR CELLS: (RODS OF CORTI) (TUNNEL CELLS) Long cells which support the walls of the inner tunnel of Corti. The tunnel is formed by the articulation of the heads of the inner and outer piller cells.

PILLARS OF CORTI: (INNER AND OUTER RODS) Two rows of rod-like bodies, with the inner rods resting on the masilar membrane at an approximate sixty degree angle. The heads of the inner rods contain a hollow which holds the convex portion of the heads of the outer rods. The outer rods, rest on the outer edge of the basilar membrane at an approximate forty degree angle. The heads of the outer rods are shaped like a flat plate containing the phalangeal processes. The phalangeal processes, along with the phalangeal processes of the cells of Deiter, form the delicate net-like reticular membrane.

PINEAL BODY: A cone-shaped, gland-like portion of the epithalamus located in a depression between the pulvinar, splenium of the corppus callosum and superior colliculi.

PINNA: (AURICLE) (AURICULA) The portion of the external ear which protudes from the sides of the head. It surrounds the opening of the external auditory canal. It is formed from cartilage which is continuous with the external auditory canal and functions to collect and direct sound waves toward the middle and inner ear.

PIRIFORM: Pear-shaped.

PISIFORM: Pea-shaped

PIT: A depression, hollow, or pocket.

PITCH INCREASE: Increase in pitch is accomplished by the changes in the length and tension of the true vocal folds. This is accomplished through the use of three intrinsic laryngeal muscles, the cricothyroid, thyroarytenoid, and posterior cricoarytenoid. The contraction of the pars recta portion of the cricothyroid muscle decreases the distance between the thyroid and cricoid cartilages anteriorly, and increases the distance between the arytenoid and thyroid cartilages. With the contraction of the pars oblique portion of the cricothyroid muscle, the thyroid cartilage slides forward on the cricoid cartilage, increasing the distance below the arytenoid and thyroid cartilages.

PITCH LEVEL: (HABITUAL LEVEL) (NATURAL LEVEL) The laryngeal tone that varies in pitch over a music range of two octaves. This level is located approximately one-fourth up the total singing range.

PITUITARY GLAND: (HYPOPHYSIS CEREBRI) A ductless gland of the endocrine system located in the sella turcica of the sphenoid bone body. It consists of the anterior and posterior lobes. The anterior lobe secretes six hormones, four of which control activities of the endocrine glands and two controlling growth and metabolism. The posterior lobe contains many nerve pathways from the hypothalamus, the major life regulating center. A hormone (antidiuretic) (ADH) secreted by the posterior lobe is responsible for maintenance of the water balance in the body.

PIVOT JOINT: (TROCHOID) Type of diarthrodial joint which restricts movement to one axis.

PLACE THEORY: (RESONANCE THEORY) Hermann Helmholtz. Proposes that the analysis of pitch preception is a function of the cochlea along the basilar membrane. The exact sensation of a pitch depending upon the maximum stimulation of the resonators, from the base (high frequency) to the apex (low frequency) along the basilar membrane. A specific pitch causes a specific resoinator to be set into motion, as each resonator has a specific nerve fiber, analysis is within the cochlea.

PLACENTA: A cake-like spongy mass. pl. placentas.

PLACODE; A plate-like structure.

PLAIN MUSCLE: (CARDIAC: SMOOTH: UNSTRIATED MUSCLE) (INVOL-UNTARY MUSCLE) Muscle, which is not under conscious control, consisting of spindly-shaped cells arranged parallel and grouped into bundles, layers, or sheets without the cross striations of other kinds of muscle. It is found in blood vessels and respiratory passages.

PLANE: A flat, smooth surface either tangent to the body, or dividing it.

PLASMA: Fluid portion of blood during circulation.

PLATE: A flattened part. Especially a flattened part of a bone.

PLATYSMA: A plate-like muscle.

PLATYSMA MUSCLE: A superficial thin muscle of the face. ORIGIN-Fascia of the cervical region over the pectoralis major, and trapezis muscles. DIRECTION- Upward. INSERTION- Mandible bone. ACTION-Depress jaw. NERVE- Facial (VII cranial) cervical branch.

PLETHYSOMOGRAPH: An instrument for determining and recording variations in air or blood volumn in organs or tissues.

PNEUMOTHORAX: The amount of air or gas in the pleural cavity which may occur either deliberately or spontaneously.

PLEURA: Delicate serous membrane that cover the lungs, walls of the diaphragm and thorax. The parietal and visceral are completely separate and are moistened with a serous secreation that reduces friction during respiratory movements of the lungs. pl. pleurae.

PLEURAL CAVITY: The space, or potential space between the parietal and visceral pleurae.

PLEURAL SINUSES: Spaces along the inferior and lower portion of the lung, which the lung does not fill.

PLEXUS: A concentration, or network of parts of the nervous and vascular system. pl. plexues.

PLICA: A fold or ridge. 2. Small folds found on the hard palate directed across midline behind the incisor teeth.

PLOSIVE: A complete stop of air that consists of a closure. Stop and release of air by the articulators.

PNEODYNAMICS: The action or dynamics of breathing.

PNEUMOGRAPH: An instrument for recording the movements of the thorax during respiration.

PNEUMOTHORAX: The presence of gas or air in the pleural cavity.

POCKET: A blind sac or cavity.

POGONION: The most anterior point of the chin at midline.

POINT OF THE CHIN: (CHIN) (MENTAL PROTUBERANCE) A triangular projection formed by the dividing of the midline ridge (mental symphysis) near the lower border of the mandible bone.

POLYMORHIC CELL: Cells appearing in many forms during different stages of development.

PONS: A process of tissue connecting parts of an organ. pl pontes.

PONS: (BRIDGE) A swelling of fibers on the brain stem ventral surface between the midbrain cerebral peduncles and medulla oblongata. It contains fiber tracts and from its border the abducent (XI cranial), auditory (VIII cranial), facial (VII cranial) and trigeminal (V cranial) nerves have their origin.

PORE: A small opening on the surface.

POSTCENTRAL GYRUS: On the parietal lobe between the central and postcentral sulci.

POSTERIOR: Toward the back, away from the front.

POSTERIOR AURICULAR NERVE: A motor and sensory branch of the facial (VII cranial) nerve. Directed to the auricularis, posterior, and occipitalis muscle, and the skin of the external auditory canal.

POSTERIOR CENTRAL GYRUS: A gyrus on the border of the central sulcus containg sensory nerve cells.

POSTERIOR COLUMN: (DORSAL HORN) (POSTERIOR HORN) The gray matter of the spinal cord which projects longer and thiner than the ventral horn. It contains sensory cells which receive and relay impulses from the fibers of the spinal nerves for receptor and co-ordination functions.

POSTERIOR COMMISSURE: A rounded bundle of white fibers of the epilhalamus. Crosses from one side of the cerebrum to the other midline at the aqueduct and third ventricle junction.

POSTERIOR CRICOARYTENOID: (CRICOARYTENOID MUSCLE) A broad intrinsic abductor muscle of the larynx. ORIGIN- The posterior portion of the cricoid cartilage. DIRECTION- Upward and lateral. INSERTION- Arytenoid cartilage muscular process, ACTION- Rotation and separation of the vocal folds. NERVE- Vagus (X cranial) laryngeal and recurrent branches.

POSTERIOR FUNICULUS: The white substance of the spinal cord. Located on each side between the dorsal root and posterior medial sulcus.

POSTERIOR HORN: (POSTERIOR COLUMN) (DORSAL HORN) The gray matter of the spinal cord which projects longer and thiner than the ventral horn. It contains sensory cells which receive and relay impulses from the fibers of the spinal nerves for receptor and co-ordination functions.

POSTERIOR INFERIOR NASAL BRANCHES: Sensory branches of the pterygopalatine nerves, a branch of the maxillary nerve, the second division of the trigeminal (V cranial) nerve. Directed to the inferior nasal concha and inferior and middle passages.

POSTERIOR INTERMEDIUS SULCUS: (DORSAL INTERMEDIATE SULCUS) Located between the dorsal lateral, and dorsal median sulci. The separation between the cuneatus and fasciculus gracilis.

POSTERIOR LATERAL SULCUS: (DORSAL LATERAL SULCUS) A long slight furrow which subdivides the spinal cord posterior portion.

POSTERIOR LIGAMENT OF THE INCUS BONE: A short, thick fibrous band connecting the short crus of the incus (anvil) bone to the fossa incudis in the tympanic cavity (middle ear).

POSTERIOR MEDIAL SEPTUM: (DORSAL MEDIAN SEPTUM) A thin

sheet of tissue which divides the spinal cord posterior portion into halves.

POSTERIOR NASAL SPINE: A sharp process forming the horizontal portion of the palatine bone.

POSTERIOR PILLAR OF FAUCES: (PALATOPHARYNGEAL ARCH) The posterior one of the two folds of mucous membrane. Formed by the downward curve from the soft palate to the side of the tongue. It encloses the palatopharyngeal muscle.

POSTERIOR SUPERIOR ALVEOLAR NERVE BRANCHES: Sensory branches of the maxillary nerve, the second division of the trigeminal (V cranial) nerve. Directed to the gingivae (gums), cheek, and molar teeth.

POSTERIOR SUPERIOR NASAL BRANCHES: Sensory nerve branches of the pterygopalatine nerves, a branch of the maxillary nerve, the second division of the trigeminal (V cranial) nerve. Directed to the ethmoid sinus, and middle and superior nasal conchea.

POSTERIOR WALL: (MASTOID WALL) Forms the posterior portion of the tympanic cavity (middle ear), and is wider above than below. It contains the enterance to the tympanic antrum, pyramidal eminence and fossa incudis.

POTASSIUM: A metallic element of the alkali group, being a soft silver white metal. Symbol: K.

POUPART'S LIGAMENT: (INGUINAL LIGAMENT) Francois Poupart, French Anatomist. A thin fibrous band of aponeurosis which joins superiorly with the lower portion of the pectoratis major muscle, the sternum bone ensiform process, and inferiorly to the anterior iliac spine and pubic symphysis.

PRECENTRAL GYRUS: The convolution on the frontal lobe extending from the lateral sulcus to the hemisphere superior margin, located between the central and precentral sulci. The area is important to the motor pathway of the skeletal muscles.

PRECUNEUS: A convolution on the medial surface of the parietal lobe, square shaped, bounded on the anterior by the paracentral lobe, and on the posterior by the medial portion of the parietooccipital sulcus.

PREMAXILLA: (INCISIVE BONE) (INTERMAXILLARY BONE) A bone formed by the median anterior portion of the superior maxilla bone by a thin suture. Consists of the floor of the anterior nasal spine and nose, and contains sockets for the incisor teeth.

PREMOLAR (BICUSPID) A tooth located distal to the canine teeth, one on each side of each jaw. Each has a two cusp crown and a cone-shaped root. Approximate eruption: permanent; 1st 9-10 years, 2nd 9-10 years.

PRESPHENOID: The anterior portion of the sphenoid bone body.

PRESSURE: Strain or stress exerted by compression, pull, thrust, or shear.

PRESSURE: Force per unit area. When force acts at right angles to a given surface, expressed as:

$$\text{Pressure} = \frac{\text{Force}}{\text{Area over which force acts}} \text{ or } P = \frac{F}{A}$$

PRESSURE-VOLUMN DIAGRAM OF BREATHING: A graph showing the relationship between the elastic and muscular forces and a column of air in the lungs.

PRIMARY BRAIN VESICLES: In embryo development, the development of the neural tube into three primary divisions; mesencephalon, prosencephalon, and rhombencephalon.

PRIMARY MOVERS: Muscles directly responsible for making desired movements.

PRIMARY TISSUE: The five basic types of body tissue; connective, epithelial, muscular, nervous and vascular.

PRIMITIVE NERVE CELL: In embryo development, a cell from the neural crest or neural tube giving off a neuron.

PRIMITIVE NODE: (HENSEN'S NODE) In embryo development, a group of cells at the cephalic end of the primary groove from which the notochord developes.

PRIMITIVE PLATE: In embryo development formed by the fusion of the nasal and maxillary processes in the stomodeum roof.

PRIMITIVE STREAK: In embryo development, the thickened, en-longated band of cells. the caudal end of the embryo dish. The first sign of germ layer development.

PRIMORDIAL: The first formed.

PRIMORDIUM: (ANALAGE) The earliest accumulation of cells in embryo development. This constitutes the beginning of a furture part, organ, or tissue.

PROCERUS: Long, slender.

PROCERUS MUSCLE: A small triangular muscle of the nose. ORIGIN- The skin over the superior portion of the nose. DIRECTION- Upward. INSERTION- Skin of the forehead at midline. ACTION- Pulls the eyebrows down. NERVE- Facial (VII cranial) buccal branch.

PROCESS: A prominence, or projection.

PROCHORDAL PLATE; In embryo development, an area of endoderm and ectoderm which developes into the pharyngeal membrane.

PROCTODEUM: In embryo development, a depression which ruptures and forms the anal canal.

PROGENITOR: An ancestor in the direct line; a parent.

PROGESTERONE: Hormone which initiates the menstrual cycle of the female.

PROLABIUM: The complete central portion of the upper lip.

PROLIFERATE: To grow by mulitiplication, as in cell division.

PROGLOSSIS: The tip of the tongue.

PROMINENCE OF THE FACIAL CANAL: A plate of bone on the medial wall of the middle ear cavity (tympanic cavity) under which the facial (VII cranial) nerve passes.

PROMONTORY: A hollow, rounded prominence formed by the first turn of the cochlea projecting into the middle ear cavity.

PRONE: Lying face down.

PROPHASE: The first phase in mitosis (cell division), when the chromatids become shorter and thicker, and the nucleoli decrease in size and disappear.

PROPRIOCEPTOR: Nerve terminals that give sensory information. Found in connective tissue, muscle spindles, and tissue.

PROSENCEPHALON: In embryo development, the anterior primitive cerebral vesicle (the forebrain) which divides into the diencephalon and telencephalon.

PROTOPLASM: Basic material in which life is processed. Composed of carbohydrates, lipins, inorganic salts, and proteins.

PROTOPLASMIC ASTROCYTE: An adult neuroglia cell with a large nucleus, abundant cytoplasm, and many expansions.

PROTUBERANCE: A knob-like projection.

PROXIMAL: Toward the point of attachment. 2. Toward the midline.

PSEUDOGLOTTIS: The opening between the false vocal folds.

PTERYGOID: Wing-shaped.

PTERYGOIDEUS MUSCLE: (INTERNAL PTERYGOID MUSCLE) A thick muscle of mastication. ORIGIN- Lateral pterygoid plate and tuber-osity of the maxilla bone. DIRECTION- Downward, lateral and back-ward. INSERTION- Mandible bone ramus medial surface and angle. ACTION- Closes the jaw. NERVE- Trigeminal (V cranial) mandibular division.

PTERYGOIDEUS LATERALIS MUSCLE: (EXTERNAL PTERYGOID MUSCLE) A thick cone-shaped muscle of mastication. ORIGIN- From two heads; the lower or inferior from the pterygoid plate lateral surface and the upper or superior from the sphenoid bone great wing. DIR-ECTION- Backward and horizontal. INSERTION- Mandible bone condyle. ACTION- Moves mandible bone side to side, opens jaws, protudes jaw. NERVE- Trigeminal (V cranial) mandible branch.

PTERYGOID CANAL: (PHARYNGEAL CANAL) Serves for transmission of the pterygoid nerves and vessels. It runs forward through the base of the sphenoid bone medial pterygoid plate, opening inferior and medial to the foramen rotundum.

PTERYGOID FOSSA: A space between the lateral and medial pterygoid plates of the sphenoid bone. The fossa contains the pterygoideus, medialis, and tensor veli palatine muscles.

PTERYGOID PROCESS: A lateral and medial plate, with the anterior portion fused, projecting downward from where the body and great wing of the spenoid bone join.

PTERYGOMANDIBULAR LIGAMENT: (PTERYGOMANDIBULAR RAPHE) A thin ridge between the buccinator and constrictor pharyngis superior muscles. It is attached inferiorly to the hyoid line of the mandible bone, and superiorly to the pterygoid hamulus.

PTERYGOPALATINE NERVE: A sensory branch of the maxillary nerve, the second division of the trigeminal (V cranial) nerve. It further divides into the greater palatine nerve directed to the soft palate, tonsil and uvula; orbital branches directed to the periosteum near the orbit and ethmoidal sphenoidal sinuses; posterior inferior nasal branches directed to the inferior nasal concha and the inferior and middle nasal passage; posterior superior nasal branches directed to the middle and superior nasal conchae and ethmoid sinuses, pharyngeal branch suppling the auditory (Eustachian) tube.

PTERYGOPALATINE SULCUS: The groove on the palatine bone perpendiculat plate forming the canal for passage of the greater palatine nerve.

PTYALIN: An enzyme containing saliva which converts starch into dextrose and maltose.

PUBERTY: The beginning of sexual maturity.

PUBIC BONE: (OS PUBIS) The anterior portion of the os coxae) on each side which articulates at midline, the pubic symphysis.

PUBIC SYMPHYSIS: The joint formed of thick cartilage at midline by the pubic bones.

PUDENDAL PLEXUS: Consists of the second, third and fourth sacral nerves which supply organs of the lower trunk.

PULMONARY: Pertaining to the lungs.

PULP: The soft portion in the center cavity of a tooth. Composed of connective tissue and containing nerves and vessels.

PULP CAVITY: The center chamber in the tooth crown.

PULVINAR: The cushion-like, medial portion of the posterior end of the thalamus. This projects medial and posteriorly over the midbrain.

PULMONARY PLEURA: (VISCERAL PLEURA) The pleura which surrounds the lungs, lines the fissures, and separates the lobes.

PUNCTIFORM: Shaped like a point.

PURE TONE: A tone which consists of only one frequency, and contains no harmonics or overtones. Described only by its frequency and intensity.

PURKINJE CELLS: Johannes E. von Purkinje, Hungarian Physiologist. Large cell bodies with dendrites extending to the cerebellar cortex and into the cerebellum white matter. The axons of these cells synapse with cells in the cerebellar nuclei.

PUTAMEN: The large dark, lateral portion of the lentiform nucleus which divides it by the lateral medullary lamina from the globus pallidus.

PYRAMID: A prominence of the medulla oblongata. Consists of motor fibers which decussate, and form the spinal cord lateral and ventral corticospinal tract.

PYRAMID OF POLYFUNCTION: An area containing the functions of breathing, deglutition, facial expression, mastication, and speech. The vertical boundry is from the ensiform process of the sternum bone to the nose tip and horizontally to the outer ear external canal.

PYRAMIDAL CELLS: Pyramid-shaped nerve cells in the cerebral cortex with attached fibers.

PYRAMIDAL DECUSSATION: Fibers of the medulla oblongata in the pyramid portion, which cross at midline and form the spinal cord lateral corticospinal tract.

PYRAMIDAL EMINENCE: Located behind the fenestra vestibuli (oval window) and in front of the vertical portion of the facial canal. It is hollow, containing the stapedius muscle. The top portion contains a small opening through which courses the tendon of the stapedius muscle.

PYRAMIDAL PATHWAY: (CORTICOSPINAL SYSTEM) PYRAMIDAL TRACT) Either of the three decending tracts of the spinal cord.

PYRAMIDAL PROCESS-PALATINE BONE: A process which forms the pterygoid fossa, projectint vertically downward, backward, and laterally from the posterior margin of the palatine bone.

PYRIFORM SINUS: A pear-shaped depression lateral to the enterance to the larynx vestibule. Bounded laterally by the thyroid cartilage, thyrophoid membrane, and medially by the aryepiglottic fold.

PYSCHOGENIC: Originating in the mind.

Q

QUADRANGULAR MEMBRANE: The upper portion of the elastic membrane of the larynx. The origin of the two portions of the membrane are from the lateral margins of the epiglottis and thyroid cartilage, moving downward to attach to the medial surfaces of the arytenoid and corniculate cartilages.

QUADRATUS LABII INFERIOR MUSCLE: (DEPRESSOR LABII INFERIOR MUSCLE) A flat small muscle of the mouth for facial expression. ORIGIN- Mandible bone lower border. DIRECTION- Lateral. INSERTION- Skin of the lower lip, and orbicularis oris muscle. ACTION- Depress lip downward. NERVE- Facial (VII cranial) buccal branch.

QUADRATUS LABII SUPERIOR MUSCLE: (LEVATOR LABII SUPERIOR MUSCLE) A triangular muscle of the mouth for facial expression with its origin from three heads.
I Angular head-
ORIGIN- Maxilla bone, frontal process. DIRECTION- Downward, lateral. INSERTION- Cartilage of the nostril and orbicularis oris muscle. ACTION Dilates the nostril, raise upper lip. NERVE- Facial (VII cranial).
II Infraorbital Head-
ORIGIN- Orbit lower margin. DIRECTION- Downward, converging. INSERTION- Orbicularis oris muscle. ACTION- Raise upper lip. NERVE- Facial (VII cranial).
III Zygomatic Head-
ORIGIN- Zygomatic bone, malar surface. DIRECTION- Downward, medial. INSERTION- Orbicularis oris muscle. ACTION- Raise upper lip. NERVE- Facial (VII cranial).

QUADRATUS LUMBORUM: A muscle of the thorax. ORIGIN- A aponeurosis from the iliac crest and the iliolumbar ligament. DIRECTION- Upward. INSERTION- Lumbar vertebrae one through four and lower border of the last rib. ACTION- Flex lumbar vertebrae. NERVE- Lumbar one through four and the thelfth thoracic.

QUADRIGEMINA: (TECTUM) The dorsal portion of the midbrain. Consisting of the inferior and superior portions.

QUADRILATERAL: A plane figure having four sides and four angles.

R

RADIAN: An angle at the center of a circle subtending its arc, and equal in length to the radius of the circle. Equal to 57.295^0.

RADIATING MUSCLE: Bundles of muscle fibers convergeing in a fan shape, decreaasing the range of motion but giving a power increase.

RADIOGRAPHY: A photograph made by the projecting roentgen (X-rays) through a portion of the body into a sensitive film.

RAMUS: A branch of an artery, vein, or nerve. 2. A bone process projecting like a branch. pl. rami.

RAMUS-MANDIBLE BONE: A quadrilateral shaped plate directed perpendicular, extending upward from the posterior portion of the mandible bone body.

RAMUS MENINGEUS: (NERVOUS SPINOSUS) A sensory branch of the mandibular nerve, the third and largest division of the trigeminal (V cranial) nerve. Directed to the dura mater and mastoid air cells.

RAPHE: A seam, or ridge indivating the line of junction of two halves.

RAREFACTION: The portion of a sound wave when air particles separate from each other.

RATE: The frequency or speed of the occurance of time, or other known standard.

RECEPTOR: A cell or group of cells that receive stimuli. 2. A sense organ.

RECESS: A small cavity or space.

RECESSUS EPITYMPANICUS: (ATTIC) (EPITYMPANIC RECESS) The superior portion of the tympanic cavity (middle ear) above the typanic membrane (eardrum) containing the malleus (hammer) bone head and the incus (anvil) bone short limb.

RECTUS: Pertaining to anything having a straight course.

RECTUS ABDOMINIS MUSCLE: A abdominal muscle of exhalation. ORIGIN- Pubis symphysis. DIRECTION- Vertical upward. INSERTION- Sternum bone enisform process and portions of ribs five through seven. ACTION- Compress the abdomen. NERVE- Intercostal.

RECURRENT: Returning to, or directed toward the origin.

RECURRENT NERVE: A motor and sensory branch of the vagus (X cranial) nerve. The left and right portions originate below the larynx, then are directed upward to supply the intrinsic muscles of the larynx, except the cricothyroid muscle, and the esophagus and trachea muscles.

RECURVE: To bend backward.

RED NUCLEUS: A mass of gray matter extending into the posterior portion of the subthalamus region. It receives fibers from the superior cerebellar peduncle.

REFLECTED WAVE: A sound wave that has been thrown back.

REFLEX: An involuntary relatively invariable adaptive response to a stimulus.

REFLEX CENTER: A center in the brain or spinal cord where sensory impressions are synapsed into a motor impulse or reflex arc.

REFRACTORY PERIOD: The time period it takes a muscle to return to its normal relaxed condition.

REGISTER: The range of pitch in voice for which the mode of vibration of the vocal folds is relatively the same, except for frequency of vibration.

REISSNER'S MEMBRANE:(VESTIBULAR MEMBRANE) Ernest Reissner, German, Anatomist. A fragile membrane which separates the scala media (cochlea duct) from the scala vestibuli and forms the roof of the cochlea duct.

RELAXATION PERIOD: The time period in which a muscle returns to a relaxed condition.

RELAXATION PRESSURE: Intrapulmonic pressure due to tissue elasticity, torque and gravity, which tends to expel air from the lungs.

REMAK FIBERS: (GRAY FIBERS) (NAKED FIBERS) Robert Remak, German Neurologist. Unmyelinated nerve fibers in the gray matter of the brain and spinal cord with the majority found in the autonomic nervous system.

RENIFORM: Kidney-shaped.

RESERVE AIR: (EXPIRATORY RESERVE VOLUME) (SUPPLEMENTAL AIR) The amount of air that can be forcible exhaled after a normal exhalation.

RESIDUAL: The remainder. 2. That which cannot be exacuated or discharged, such as residual air in the lungs.

RESIDUAL AIR: The amount of air remaining in the lungs after the fullest possible expiration.

RESONANCE: The intensification of sound. Produced by the communication of a vibration to an external sound.

RESONATING CAVITIES: Consists of the mouth cavity, paranasal sinuses, pharynx, and superior portion of the larynx.

RESPIRATION: The act of breathing. 2. To draw and expell air from the lungs.

RESPIRATORY PASSAGE: The bronchial tubes, larynx, nares, nasal cavities, oral cavity, pharynx, and trachea.

RESTIFORM: Shaped like a rope.

RESTIFORM BODY: (INFERIOR CEREBELLAR PEDUNCLES) Afferent fibers connecting the cerebellum and medulla oblongata. Also forms the fourth ventricle lateral wall.

RETICULAR: Fibers, lines, or veins criss-crossing. 2. A network of such fibers. 3. Fibers passing between the pons and the medulla oblongata.

RETICULAR FORAMATION: (SPINAL FORMATION) Gray matter located between the dorsal and lateral horns in the spinal cord. Directs thin projections into the white matter, giving a net-like appearance.

RETICULAR LAMINA: A very delicate framework perofrated and filled by the free end of the outer hair cells.

RETICULAR MEMBRANE: A net-like membrane over the organ of Corti with the free ends of the outer hair cells passing through the opening. It is formed by the heads of the inner rods, inner phalanges, phalangeal, process of the outer rods, and the heads of the Deiter's cells.

RETICULAR TISSUE: Type of connective tissue containing delicate fibers that form an interlacing network. It provides support for lymph nodes. It is found in the bone marrow, liver, lungs, muscle tissue, and spleen.

RETRACT: Draw back, or shorten.

RETROLINGUAL: Behind the tongue.

REUNIENS DUCT: (CANAL REUNIEN) (DUCT OF HENSEN) A membranous short tube from the scala media (cochlea duct) to the saccula in the vestibule of the inner ear which allows endolymph fluid interchange.

RHEOBASE: The minimum strength of electric current necessary to produce stimulation of a nerve.

RHOMBENCEPHALON: (HINDBRAIN) In embryo development, the hindbrain which divides into the metencephalon and myelencephalon. Includes the cerebellum, medulla oblongata, and pons.

RHOMBIC LIP: In embryo development, the lateral boundary of the rhombencephalon where the floor plate bends. Here the lip forms which fuses with the alar lamina coverning the trigeminal (V cranial) nerve.

RHOMBOID: Shaped like a kite.

RIB: One bone of a set of twelve pair which are curbed and narrow. Extends anteriorly and laterally from the sides of the thorax vertebrae by costal cartilages, except for rib pairs eleven and twelve.

RIB ANGLE: The point where the direction of the rib abruptly changes.

RIB CAGE: (THORACIC CAVITY) The steletal framework of the chest. Consists of the ribs (twelve pair of flat long curved bones), sternum bone, and thoracic vertebrae.

RIB MOVEMENT: For inhalation, the thoracic cavity increases on the anterior-posterior diameter by forward and upward movement of the sternum bone. The tranverse diameter increases by the raising of the ribs, and the vertical diameter is increased by cintraction of the diaphragm.

RIB SHAFT: The somewhat flat, major portion of the rib.

RIBONUCLEIC ACID: A nucleic acid found in all living cell nucleolus, microsomes, and mitochondria. It is a catalyst for the production of protein and responsible for information transfer from DNA (deoxyribonucleic acid) to the cell protein system. Abbreviation: RNA.

RIDGE: An elevation or crest.

RIMA: A cleft or crack. pl. rimae.

RIMA GLOTTIDIS: (FISSURE OF GLOTTIS) (GLOTTAL CHINK) An enlongated fissure between the true vocal folds in front, and the bases and the vocal ligaments of the arytenoid cartilages behind. Its shape and width depend on the arytenoid cartilages and true vocal folds during phonation and respiration. The anterior membranous portion, approximately three fifths the length, is the membranous (vocal) glottis bounded laterally by the muscular portion of the vocal folds. It extends from the anterior commissure of the true vocal folds to the vocal process of the arytenoid cartilages. The cartilaginous glottis is the posterior portion and is bounded by the vocal processes and medial surfaces of the arytenoid cartilages. The length, width, and shape, of the glottis differs from person to person.

RIMA VESTIBULI: (FLASE GLOTTIS) The space between the left and right vestibular folds of the larynx.

RISORIUS MUSCLE: A muscle of the mouth and of facial expression. ORIGIN- Fascia over the masseter muscle. DIRECTION- Horizontal and forward. INSERTION- Skin, at the angle of the mouth. ACTION- Pulls mouth angle lateral. NERVE- Facial (VII cranial) mandibular and buccal branches.

RIVINUS LIGAMENT: (PARS FLACCIDA) (SHRAPNELL'S MEMBRANE) A small triangular portion of the tympanic membrane (ear drum) in the superior portion which fills the notch of Rivinus. It is less tense than the rest of the ear drum.

RNA: Abbreviation for ribonucleic acid.

RODS OF CORTI: (PILLAR CELLS) (TUNNEL CELLS) Long cells which support the walls of the inner tunnel of Corti. The tunnel is formed by the articulation of the heads of the inner and outer pillar cells.

ROOF: (TEGMEN TYMPANI) (TEGMENTAL WALL) The roof, formed by a thin layer of the temporal bone petrous portion, over the tympanic cavity (middle ear) separating it from the meninges of the cranium.

ROOF OF THE MOUTH: (PALATE) A bony plate separating the nasal and oral cavities. It consists of a hard palate in front and a soft palate behind. It functions to change the degree of coupling between the nasopharynx and vocal tract.

ROOT: Portion of a tooth implanted in the gingiva (gum) tissue covered by cementum.

ROSENMULLER'S FOSSA: (PHARYNGEAL RECESS) Johann C. Rosenmuller, German Physician. A depression in the wall of the pharynx, above and behind the auditory (Eustachian) tube.

ROOT: (BASE) The portion of the tongue connected to the hyoid bone by the hyoglossal membrane and genioglossus and hyoglossus muscles, and to the epiglottis by the glossoepiglottic mucous membrane, the soft palate by the glossopalatine arches, and the constrictor pharyngis superior muscle.

ROSTRAD: (CRANIAL) (CEPHALAD) Toward the head. 2. The front or superior portion of the body.

ROSTRAL: Having a beak.

ROSTRUM: (SPHENOIDAL ROSTRUM) A ridge on the sphenoid bone inferior surface which articulates with a depression between the vomer bone wings.

ROUND WINDOW: (FENESTRA ROTUNDA) A round opening into the base turn of the scala tympani of the cochlea. It is located in the labrinthic wall under the fenestra vestibuli (oval window) in a funnel shaped depression hidden by the promontory. The opening is closed by a thin membrane, the secondary tympanic membrane.

RUBROSPINAL TRACT: An ascending tract of the spinal cord lateral funiculus. The majority of the motor fibers originate from cells of the red nucleus of the superior colliculi.

RUDIMENTARY: Being imperfectly developed. The beginning of development.

RUGA: A wrinkle or fold. pl. rugae.

S

SAC: A baglike organ or structure. 2. A pouch that may contain fluid.

SACCULE: The smaller of the two sacs in the bony vestibule of the inner ear. It communicates with the endolymphatic duct, cochlea duct, and utricle, all filled with endolymph fluid. A sensory area, the macula acustica sacculi is in its wall. 2. A small sac.

SACCULE OF THE LARYNX: (VENTRICULAR APPENDIX) A small sac extending from the laryngeal ventricle. Located between the thyro-arytenoid muscle. and ventricular fold.

SACCURAL DUCT: (UTRICULOSACCULARIS) A duct which joins the saccule and utricle of the membranous labyrinth.

SACRAL: Pertaining to the sacrum. A somewhat triangular shaped bone, formed by the five bones that are fused and wedged dorsally, between the two hip bones.

SACRAL NERVES: The five pair of motor and sensory nerves. The first four enter the pelvis and the fifth enters between the coccyx and sacrum.

SACRAL PLEXUSES: Composed of the five pair of sacral spinal nerves which form a band, the sciatic nerve.

SACROILIAC JOINT: An articulation between the os coxae (hip bone) and sacrum. Formed by a amphiarthrodial (yielding) joint between the lateral border of the sacrum and the posterior portion of the inner surface of each ilium.

SACROSPINALIS MUSCLE: A deep intrinsic layer of the back. ORIG-IN-Iliac crest, lumbar vertebrae and sacrum. DIRECTION- Verti-cal. INSERTION- Iliocostalis and longissumus dorsi muscle. AC-TION- Extends the vertebral column. NERVE- Spinal, dorsal pri-mary division.

SACROSPINALIS MUSCLE GROUPS: Consists of three major groups: Medial Spinalis- Spinalis Captis

Spinalis Cervicis
Spinalis Dorsi (Thoracis)
Medial Longissimus- Longissimus Capitis
Longissimus Cervicis
Longissimus Dorsi (Thoracis)
Lateral Iliocostalis- Ilicostalis Cervicis
Ilicostalis Dorse (Thoracis)
Ilicostalis Lumborum

SACRUM: Triangle-shaped bone formed by five united vertebra between the fifth lumbar vertebra and the coccyx. It forms the base of the vertebral column. With the coccyx it helps form the dorsal portion of the pelvis, articulating from the sacroilioc joints.

SADDLE JOINT: Type of diarthrodial joint which permits all movements except rotation. The articular surface of each bone is concave in one direction, and convex in the other.

SAGITTAL: An anatomic plane, from front to back dividing into right and left portions. 2. Shaped like an arrow.

SALINE: A solution containing sodium chloride (salt).

SALIVA: A clear, alkaline, tasteless, secretion from the parotid, sublingual, and submaxillary mucous glands of the mouth. It moistens and softens food, and moistens the mouth. Also contains mucin, the base element, and is neutralized by the gastric juice in the stomach.

SALIVARY GLANDS: Consists of three pair; parotid, submandibular, and sublingual.

SALPINGIAN: Pertaining to the auditory tube.

SALPINGOPALATINE MUSCLE: ORIGIN- Auditory tube cartilage. DIRECTION- Downward and forward. INSERTION- Blends with the muscle of the soft palate. ACTION- Raises the nasopharynx. NERVE- Vagus (X cranial) pharyngeal plexus.

SALPINGOPALATINE FOLD; A mucous membrane from the lateral pharyngeal wall to the opening of the auditory (Eustachian) tube.

SALPINGOPHARYNGEUS MUSCLE; A pharyngeal levator muscle. ORIGIN- Near the opening of the auditory tube. DIRECTION- Downward. INSERTION- Blends with mucous membrane of the pharynx. ACTION- Raises the pharynx. NERVE Vagus (X cranial) pharyngeal plexus.

SARCOLUMMA: A delicate membrane surrounding each striated muscle fiber.

SARCOPLASM: Semifluid between fibers of striated muscle cells.

SCALA: The stairlike structure of the passages of the cochlea. 2. Any one of the spiral passages of the cochlea, the sacla media, scala tympani, or scala vestibuli.

SCALA MEDIA: (COCHLEA DUCT) (MEMBRANOUS COCHLEA) The tube triangular shaped within the cochlea separated from the scala vestibuli by Reissner's membrane and from the scala tympani by the basilar membrane. The duct contains the organ of Corti and endolymph fluid.

SCALA TYMPANI: The lower portion of the cochlea containing perilymph fluid. It extends from the fenestra rotunda (round window) to the helicotrema (tip) of the cochlea.

SCALA VESTIBULI: (VESTIBULAR CANAL) The upper portion of the cochlea contining perilymph fluid. It extends from the fenestra vestibuli (oval window) to the helicotrema (tip) of the cochlea.

SCALENE MUSCLES: Consist of the Anterior, Medius and Posterior muscle of the neck. ORIGIN- Cervical vertebrae three through six, transverse processes. DIRECTION- Downward. INSERTION- First First rib tubercle. ACTION- Flex neck, flex first rib. NERVE-Cervical plexus (four through eight).

SCALUS: Uneven. Used to name various muscles.

SCAPHA: Long, curved depression that separates the helix from the anthelix.

SCAPHOID: Shaped like a boat.

SCAPHOID FOSSA: A depression on the pterygoid process of the sphenoid bone for the tensor veli palatini muscle.

SCAPULA: (SHOULDER BLADE) A flat, thin, triangular shaped plate of bone, dorsal to ribs seven and eight, covered with muscles. It is lateral to the vertebral column on the posterior-superior wall of the rib cage. It is freely movable, articulating with the clavicle and humerus bones.

SCAPULAE NOTCH: An indentation on the superior border of the scapula bone at the coracoid process base. This is converted into a foramen by a ligament.

SCARP'S FLUID: (ENDOLYMPH) Antonio Scarpa, Italian Physician. Pale, watery fluid within the scala medial (cochlea duct) and membranous labyrinth. Secreted by the stria vascularis.

SCARP'S MEMBRANE: (SECONDARY TYMPANIC MEMBRANE) The membrane which closes the fenestra rotunda (round window) of the tympanic cavity (middle ear).

SCHINDYLESIS: Type of synarthrosis joint where a plate of bone is inserted into a cleft formed by the separation of two laminae in another bone.

SCLEROTOME: In embryo development, mesenchymal tissue on each side of the notchord which develops into the ribs and vertebrae.

SEBUM: Secretion of the sebaceous glands. A semi-thick fluid, composed of fat and epithelial debris, from the cells of the malpighiam layer.

SEBACEOUS GLANDS: Glands that secrete an oily substance, sebum.

SECOND ORDER NEURONS: Nerve fibers directed from the dorsal and ventral cochlea nuclei to the trapezoid body and lateral lemniscus in the auditory pathway.

SECONDARY PALATE: The palate proper formed by the fusion of the palatine processes of the maxilla bones.

SECONDARY TEETH: (PERMANENT TEETH) The second set of teeth which appear from approximately the sixth through the twenty-fifth year. The thirty-two teeth include two canine, four incisor, six molar and four premolar in each jaw represented by the following dental formula:

$$I \frac{2-2}{2-2} \qquad C \frac{1-1}{1-1} \qquad PM \frac{2-2}{2-2} \qquad M \frac{3-3}{3-3}$$

Approximate Eruption in Years

First molars	6-7	Second premolars	9-10
Central incisors	7-8	Canines	12-14
Lateral incisors	7-8	Second molars	12-15
First premolars	9-10	Third molars	17-25

SECONDARY TYMPANIC MEMBRANE: (SCARP'S MEMBRANE) The membrane which closes the fenestra rotunda (round window) of the tympanic cavity (middle ear).

SECTION: A segment or division of a organ or part.

SEGMENTATION: Small parts, or segments.

SELECTIVE PERMEABILITY: A membrane that permits only certain substances to pass in or out.

SELLA: A saddle shaped depression. pl. sallae.

SELLA TURCICA: A depression on the sphenoid bone superior surface crossing at midline. This contains the hypophysis (pituitary gland).

SEMICIRCULAR CANALS; The lateral, posterior, and superior canals of the inner ear situated at right angles to each other. They are filled with endolymph fluid and, along with the saccule and utricle, complete the balance organ.

SEMILUNAR: Resembling a crescent or half moon.

SEMILUNAR GANGLION: A sensory ganglion of the trigeminal (V cranial) nerve. Consists of a mass which divides into the mandibular, maxillary and ophthalmic nerve branches.

SEMILUNAR NOTCH: (MANDIBULAR NOTCH) A deep depression on the mandible bone ramus portion on the superior border. Separates the coronoid and condyloid processes.

SENSORY: Process of sensation. 2. Nerves, organs, or structures that carry stimuli from the exterior to the cerebro-spinal system.

SENSORY NERVE: Afferent nerve which carries a stimulus toward the brain or ventral nervous system.

SENSORY NEURON: A afferent neruon which communicates sensory impulses.

SENSORY ROOT: (DORSAL ROOT) Originates in the dorsal ganglion, outside the spinal cord, with a single fiber directed into two processes. One extends to the sensory end organ of a joint, muscle, or tendon and the other extending into the spinal cord to form the dorsal root.

SENSORY RECEPTOR: A cell or group of cells responding to an external stimulus.

SEPTUM: A partition between two cavities. pl. septa.

SEPTUM CANALIS MUSCULOTUBARII: A thin plate of bone dividing the musculotubal canal into the canals for the auditory tube and tensor tympani muscle.

SEPTUM PELLUCIDUM: A double membrane partition between the anterior horns of the lateral ventricles of the brain.

SEROUS: Characterized by serum.

SEROUS MEMBRANE: The membrane lining of external walls of the body cavities. The membrane consists of mesothelium (a squamous cell layer) on a layer of connective tissue which secretes watery material.

SERRATED: Notched on the edge, like a saw.

SERRATUS ANTERIOR MUSCLE: A thoracic muscle of inhalation. ORIGIN- In the form of digitations from ribs one through eight or nine. DIRECTION- Backward. INSERTION- Complete scapula vertebral border. ACTION, Fix scapula, raise ribs one through eight. NERVE- Thoracic from the brachial plexus.

SERRATUS POSTERIOR INFERIOR MUSCLE: A thoracic muscle of inhalation. ORIGIN- Spines of thoracic vertebrae eleven and twelve and lumbar vertebrae one and two. DIRECTION- Upward and lateral. ACTION- Pulls ribs back and downward. NERVE- Thoracic eleven and twelve.

SERRATUS POSTERIOR SUPERIOR MUSCLE: A thoracic muscle of inhalation. ORIGIN- Spines of cervical vertebrae six and seven and thoracic vertebrae one and two. DIRECTION- Downward and lateral. INSERTION- Angle of ribs two through five. ACTION- Raise ribs in inspiration. NERVE- Thoracic nerves one through four.

SERUM: Any watery fluid from animals.

SESAMOID: (LESSER ALAR) The cartilage forming a portion of the nasal lateral wall.

SHAFT: A long slim part. 2. A portion of a rib bone.

SHEATH: A tubular structure enclosing or surrounding muscles, nerves, or vessels.

SHEATH OF HENLE: Friedrich G. Henle, German Anatomist. A sheath of connective tissue which is between the alpha fibers and the sarcoplasm of a muscle fiber.

SHEATH OF RECTUS ABDOMINIS: A broad, flat, sheet of tendon (aponeurosis) enclosing the rectus abdominis muscle.

SHEATH OF SCHWANN: (MEDULLARY SHEATH) Theodor Schwann, German Physician. A layer of myelin which surrounds nerve fibers, and functions as an insulator.

S. H. M. : Abbreviation for simple marmonic motion.

SHORT CRUS-INCUS BONE: (SHORT PROCESS) Slighly cone-shaped and attached to the fossa incridis in the back and lower portion of the epitympanic recess.

SHOULDER: The point and junction of the arm meeting the trunk at the clavicle and scapula bones.

SHOULDER BLADE: (SCAPULA) Flat, thin triangular shaped plate of bone, dorsal to ribs seven and eight, covered with muscles. It is located lateral to the vertebral column on the posterior-superior wall of the rib cage. It is freely moveable, articulating with the clavicle and humerus bones.

SHRAPNELL'S MEMBRANE: (PARS FLACCIDA) Henry J. Shrapnell, English anatomist. The superior triangular portion of the tympanic membrane (eardrum). Located between the malleolar folds filling the notch of Rivinus.

SIBILANT: Characterized by a hissing or whistling sound.

SIGMOID: Shaped like the letter S.

SIMPLE HARMONIC MOTION: Motion produced by the tines of a tuning fork or a pendulum swinging through a arc. Projected uniform motion. Abbreviation: S. H. M.

SIMPLEX LOBULUS: The portion of the cerebellum, continuous with the declive portion of the vermis, caudal to the primary fissure.

SINE WAVE: A wave that expresses the sine of a linear function of space, time or both. It differs in amplitude, frequency or phase relationship, riseing to its crest, and falling to its trough in a regular rhythmic manner.

SINGULAR FORAMEN: An opening in the internal auditory canal for passage of the nerves to the posterior semicircular duct.

SINUS: A cavity or hollow space within a bone. Developed from the nasal cavities and lined with mucous membrane continuous with the nasal cavity. Air filled, they communicate with the nasal cavities and their minute openings. Their function is not completely understood but thought to filter, moisten and warm the air. 2. Air cavities in the facial bones. pl sinus, sinuses.

SITUS: In position or site.

SKELETAL MUSCLE: (STRIATED: STRIDED: VOLUNTARY MUSCLE) Muscle which is under conscious control consisting of fibers grouped into bundles, or fasciculi covered by a sheath of connective tissue. It is voluntary muscle which is attached to bone and is found in the pharynx, skeletal muscles, tongue and the superior portion of the esophagus.

SKIFF: A slight depression on the external ear near the entrance to the external canal.

SKIN: The outer covering of the body. This consists of the major layer of connective tissue containing lymphatics, nerves, nerve endings, and the outer layer, the epidermis.

SKULL: (CRANIUM) The bony framework of the head consisting of eight cranial bones, housing and protecting, the brain. One each of the ethmoid, frontal, occipital and sphenoid, and two each of the parietal and temporal. Fourteen facial bones for the framework for most of the speech mechanism consisting of one each of the mandible and vomer and two each of the inferior conchae, lacrimal, maxilla, nasal, palatine and zygomatic bones.

SMALL SUBLINGUAL DUCTS: (DUCTS OF RIVINUS) The ducts which drain the sublingual gland posterior portion.

SMALL WINGS- SPHENOID BONE: Two processes of thin bone from the anterior and superior portion of the body which are projected laterally. The inferior surface forms a portion of the orbit roof. The superior surface supports a portion of the brain, and the anterior border articulates with the frontal bone. They contain the optic foramen for passage of the ophthalmic artery and optic (II cranial) nerve.

SMOOTH MUSCLE: (INVOLUNTARY MUSCLE) (CARDIAC: PLAIN, UNSTRIATED) Muscle, which is not under conscious control, consisting of spindly-shaped cells arranged parallel and grouped into bundles, layers, or sheets without the cross striations of other kinds of muscle. It is found in blood vessels and respiratory passages.

SOCKET: A depression, or hollow into which another part fits.

SODIUM: A metallic element being soft, silver-white, and alkaline. Symbol, Na.

SOFT PALATE: (VELUM) A curtain-like movable fold suspended from the posterior border of the hard palate. It may be lowered, raised, or tensed by five muscles; two elecators, levator palatine and uvular, two depressor relaxors, glossopalatine and pharyngopalatine; and an elevator tensor, the tensor palatine (tensor veli palatine). The resonant characteristics of the vocal tract are modified by the lowering or raising of the palate. It is lowered for nasal sound and breathing and raised for production of vowel sounds.

SOFT PALATE MUSCLES: Consists of the glossopalatine, levator veli palatine, pharyngopalatine, tensor veli palatine, and uvula.

SOMATIC: Pertaining to the body.

SOMATIC MESODERM: In embryo development, the outer of two layers into which the mesoderm separates.

SOMATIC NERVE FIBERS: The threadlike alpha, beta, or gamma fibers of the somatic nervous system. These are involved in voluntary body activities, having conduction velocities of twenty to one hundred meters per second.

SOMATIC NERVES: The nerves directed to the skeletal muscles.

SOMATIC NERVOUS SYSTEM: The portion of the nervous system which controls the voluntary muscles.

SOMITES: In embryo development, block-like segments of mesoderm on each side of the neural tube which forms the vertebral column.

SOUND: Auditory sensations made by vibration. Measurement of sound is in decibels (dB), which is the ratio of two amounts of acoustic or electric signal power equal to ten times the logarithm of this ratio. 2, A form of vibration energy that gives auditory sensation.

SOUND PRESSURE: The change of a medium caused by the energy and force of sound.

SOUND PRESSURE LEVEL: The intensity of sound measured in decibels. Abbrivation: SPL.

SOUND PRESSURE MEASURMENT: Represented by the formula, dyne/cm^2, the dyne being the amount of energy required to impart an acceleration of one centimeter per second per second.

SOUND WAVE: Pressure of air particals in a medium set into motion in concentric spheres. They are measured as to frequency, intensity and spectrum. Sound wave frequency is determined by the frequency of vibration at the source.

SPACE: An area, cavity, or region actual or potential of the body.

SPACE OF NUEL: (NUELS SPACE) Jean P. Nuel, Belgian otologist. The space between the outer piller and outer phalangeal cells. They provide a passage for nerve fibers and endolymph fluid, which baths and nourishes the inner cells of the organ of Corti.

SPECIAL INTEROCEPTOR: A recepter for sensations of smell, taste, or thirst.

SPECIFIC GRAVITY: The ratio of the mass of a given volume of a substance to that of the same volume of some other substance. Water is the standard for liquids and solids, while air, or hydrogen is the standard for gases.

SPECTRUM: The band of colors formed when visible light is passed through a prism or other light dispersing device. In sound, a representation of the amplitude (also phase) of the components arranged as a function of their frequencies.

SPECULUM: An instrument for dilating the orifice of a cavity or tube in order that the interior may be observed.

SPEECH: The verbal expression of though by articulation of sounds.

SPEECH CENTER: (AREA44-45) (BROCA'S AREA) Pierre P. Broca,

French Surgeon. The area on the left side of the brain in the inferior frontal gyrus rostal to the motor area (area 8) for motor speech.

SPEECH PRODUCTION: Sounds produced in four phases; respiration, phonation, resonation, and articulation. Associated areas are; larynx, lungs, pharynx, nasal cavity, oral cavity (mouth), and trachea.

SPENOPALATINE GANGLION: A triangular shaped parasympathetic ganglion in the eteryqopalatine fossa which contains motor and sensory fibers. Divides into the orbital, palatine, pharyngeal, and posterior superior nasal branches.

SPERM CELL: The spermatozoon formed within the testes.

SPERMATOGENSIS; The forming of mature functional spermatozoa.

SPERMATOZOON: A mature male sperm cell consisting of the nucleus, neck, middle, and tail.

SPHENOID: Wedge shaped.

SPHENOID BONE: A single, irregular bone located at the base of the skull, anterior to the base of the occipital and temporal bones. It is bat shaped with wings fully extended, divided into the body, great and lesser wings, and pterygoid processes and also contains the sphenoid sinuses which open into the nasal passages. Articulation is with the palatine, vomer bones, and all bones of the cranium.

SPHENOID SINUSES: Cavities of various size and shape located in the anterior portion of the sphenoid bone body. They communicate with the highest passage of the nasal cavity on the same side. At birth they are tiny cavities which develope after puberty.

SPHENOIDAL FISSURE: A fissure between the great wing of the sphenoid bone and the temporal bone petrous portion.

SPHENODIAL PROCESS-PALATINE BONE: A irregular projection directed inward and medial. The concave medial portion forms a portion of the nasal cavity lateral wall.

SPHENOIDAL ROSTRUM) (ROSTRUM) A ridge on the sphenoid bone inferior surface which articulates with a depression between the vomer bone wings.

SPHENOMANDIBULAR LIGAMENT: (INTERNAL LATERAL LIGAMENT) A flat, thin band attached to the inner surface of the mandible bone ramus and the spina angularis of the sphenoid bone.

SPHENOPALATINE NOTCH: The indentation between the palatine bone oribital and sphenoid processes.

SPHINCTER: A ringlike muscle fiber that close a natural opening or passage.

SPHINCTER OF WHILLIS: (VELOPHARYNGEAL SPHINCTER MUSCLE) A portion of the superior constrictor muscle. ORIGIN- Soft palate at midline. DIRECTION- Horizontal backward. INSERTION- Pharynx median raphe. ACTION- Contracts pharynx. NERVE- Vagus (X cranial, pharyngeal plexus.

SPIDER CELL: (ASTROCYTE) A neuroglia cells, star-shaped with many branching processes.

SPIKE: The abrupt, potential change at the beginning of a nervous impulse.

SPINA: A thornlike projection or process. pl. spinae.

SPINA ANGULARIS: A bony process, small in size, directed downward from the great wing of the spenoid bone, and projecting between the petrous and squama portions of the temporal bone. The pterygospinous and sphenomandibular ligaments are attached to it.

SPINAL CANAL: Formed by the vertebrae foramina containing the spinal cord and meninges.

SPINAL COLUMN: The vertebral column enclosing the spinal cord, joined together by intervertebral cartilages and ligaments. It consists of vertebrae bones; seven cervical, twelve thoracic, five lumbar, five saccral fused together and from three to five coccygeal.

SPINAL CORD: A long, slender cylinder of gray and white matter within the vertebral column spinal canal. Extends from the occipital bone foramen magnum, downward to the level of the first lumbar vertebra. Two areas of the cord are slightly enlarged, the cervical and lumbar regions for the connection of spinal nerves directed to the upper and lower extremities. The cord ends as a tapered tip of fine filament-like fibers, the filum terminate.

SPINAL CORD-LATERAL FUNICULUS-ASCENDING TRACTS: Consists of the dorsal spinocerebeller, dorsolateral, lateral proper fasciculus, lateral spinothalamic, spinotectal and ventral spinocerebeller.

SPINAL CORD-LATERAL FUNICULUS -DECENDING TRACTS: Consists of the lateral cortiospinal, lateral reticulospinal, olivospinal and rubrospinal.

SPINAL CORD-VENTRAL FUNICULUS-ASCENDING TRACTS: Consists of the ventral proper fasciculus and ventral spinothalamic.

SPINAL CORD-VENTRAL FUNICULUS-DESCENDING TRACTS: Consist of the sulcomarginal fasciculus, tectospinal, ventral corticospinal ventral reticulospinal vestibulospinal.

SPINAL FLUID: (CEREBROSPINAL FLUID) A clear fluid covering the brain and spinal cord. The fluid is produced by highly vascular folds or processes (choroid plexuses) of the pia mater layer in the ventricles and functions as a fluid shock absorber and nutritive for nerve cells.

SPINAL FORMATION: (RETICULAR FORMATION) Gray matter, located between the dorsal and lateral horns in the spinal cord, directing thin projections into the white matter giving a net-like appearance.

SPINAL GANGLION: Oval shaped enlargement of the spinal nerve dorsal root.

SPINAL NERVES: Consists of thirty one pair of nerves which arise from the spinal cord in the spinal canal. They are directed through the intervertebral foramina and emerge as dorsal (sensory-afferent) and ventral (motor efferent) roots. They are divided as: eight cervical, (C1 thru C-8 directed horizontal); twelve thoracic(T1 thru T12 directed downward); Five lumbar (L1 thru L5 directed vertical); five sacral (S1 thru S5 directed vertical); and one coccygeal.

SPINAL PART-ACCESSORY NERVE: A motor portion of the accessory (XI cranial) nerve. Its origin is in the spinal cord as roots for cervical nerves one through five. These are directed through the the jugular foramen to supply the sternocleidomastoid and trapezius muscles.

SPINAL ROOT: A portion of the spinal nerve with the motor portions being the ventral roots, and the sensory portion being the dorsal roots.

SPINDLE: A structure appearing in the metaphase of mitosis (cell division). Consists of a bundle of fibrils which connect the two centrosomes.

SPINDLE CELL: A fusiform, or spindle-shaped cell.

SPINE: A thorn-like projection or process. 2. A sharp process of bone.

SPINE: (BACKBONE) (VERTEBRAL COLUMN) A portion of the axial skeleton from the coccyx through the cranium. Consists of the coccyx, sacrum, five lumbar, twelve thoracic, and seven cervical vertebrae, enclosing and protecting the spinal cord.

SPINOTECTAL TRACT: An ascending tract of the spinal cord. Located ventral to the lateral spinothalamic tract in the lateral lemniscus, and terminating in the superior colliculus.

SPINOUS PROCESS: A projection at the posterior part of each vertebra.

SPIRAL: Winding around a center, like a coil or the threads of a screw.

SPIRAL CANAL OF THE MODIOUS: (CANAL OF ROSENTHAL) Isidor Rosenthal, German Physiologist. A passage containing the spiral ganglion of the cochlear division of the auditory (VIII cranial) nerve which follows the direction of the osseous spiral lamina of the inner ear.

SPIRAL GANGLION: The ganglion located in the modiolus of the inner ear. Consists of the central processes, forming the cochlear portion of the acoustic (VIII cranial) nerve, and the peripheral processes terminating in the organ of Corti.

SPIRAL LAMINA: A bony ledge, or shelf consisting of two very thin plates of bone between which canals for transmission of the acoustic nerve fibers are located. It projects from the modiolus into the cochlea canal, partially dividing it into the lower portion the scala tympani and the upper portion the scala vestibuli. It is narrow at the apex end, widing toward the basal end.

SPIRAL LIGAMNET: The thick portion of the lining of the bony cochlea. Projects inward forming the outer wall of the cochlea duct, to which the outer edge of the basilar membrane attaches.

SPIRAL LIMBUS: A thick portion of the bony spiral lamina. The outer edge is concave to form a spiral sulcus dividing into a lower tympanic lip and upper vestibular lip.

SPIRAL ORGAN OF CORTI: (ORGAN OF CORTI) Alfonso Corti,
Italian Anatomist. The recepter, sensory, transmitter system of
the ear, located in the cochlea and resting on the basilar membrane.
It consists of hair cells and rod-shaped cells which extend into
the endolymph fluid of the scala medial(cochlea duct). Projecting
over the cells from the spiral lamina is a roof-like coverning, the
tectorial membrane. Attached to the membrane are the hairs of the
cell so that through vibration of the basilar membrane the hair cells
relax and stretch. The auditory nerve (VIII cranial) cochlea nerve
branch contains fibers arising in the spiral ganglion nerve cells
from the modiolus. These are directed to the brain, some end in
the organ hair cells, and others around the hair cells of the organ
of Corti.

STRIA VASCULARIS: A layer of highly vascular pigmented granular
cells on the outer wall of the cochlear duct.

SPIROMETER: Instrument for measuring the air taken into and exhaled from the lungs.

SPIROID: Resembling a spiral.

SPL: Abbrivation for sound pressure level, the intensity of sound
measured in decibels (dB).

SPLANCHNIC MESODERM: In embryo development, the inner of the
two layers into which the mesoderm separates.

SPLANCHNOLOGY: The study of the body viscera.

SPLENIUM: A structure with a handlike shape.

SPONGIFORM: Resembling a sponge.

SPONGIOBLAST: Cells developing from the embryo neural tube which
change into astrocutes and ependymal cells.

SPONGY BONE: (CANCELLOUS BONE) Bone substance of thin intersecting lamellae of bars and plates. Forms many connunicating
spaces filled with bone marrow in the interior of a bone.

SQUAMA: Platelike structure or scale.

SQUAMA-FRONTAL BONE: The convex portion of the frontal bone
forming the forehead. Usually presenting at midline a frontal or

metopic suture which is present at birth, dividing the bone in two.

SQUAMA PORTION- OCCIPITAL BONE: The largest of the three portions extending from the posterior edge of the opening of the magnum foramen to the lambdoid suture. Appearing rough, the uneven external surface contains a prominence, the external occipital protuberance. Extending laterally from the occipital protuberance are two curved ridges, the higher and superior nuchal lines. Articulation is with the parietal and temporal bones.

SQUAMOUS CELLS: Flat, scalelike epithelial cells.

SQUAMOUS PORTION-TEMPORAL BONE: Forming the anterior and superior portion of the temporal bone. An extremely thin translucent bone from the inferior portion of the zygomatic process. It projects with the anterior end for articulation with the zygomatic bone temporal process.

SQUAMOUS SUTURE: (SQUAMOSAL SUTURE) The junction of the parietal and temporal bones squamous portions.

STANDING WAVE: Produced by the interference of two periodic sound waves of the same amplitude and frequency traveling in opposite directions. The amplitude doubles at some points and is zero at others. The wave is reflected back, without a phase change setting up the pattern of amplitude cancellations and reinforcements.

STAPEDIS CAPITULUM: The stapes (stirrus) bone head which articulates with the incus (anvil) bone.

STAPEDIUS MUSCLE: A muscle of the tympanic cavity (middle ear). ORIGIN- Interior of pyramid eminence. DIRECTION-vertical and horizontal. INSERTION-Posterior surface of the stapes bone neck. ACTION- Pulls down and posterior on stapes footplate. NERVE-Facial (VII cranial) tympanic branch.

STAPES BONE-BASE: A flat, oval plate which forms the footplate of the stapes bone fitting into the fenestra vestibuli (oval window) with a fiberous ring.

STAPES BONE: (STIRRUP) The third and inner most bone of the ossicles of the tympanic cavity (middle ear). It articulates with the incus (anvil) bone, and the stapes footplate inserts into the fenestra vestibuli (oval window). It consists of the head, neck, footplate, and two crus (legs).

STAPES HEAD: A concave facet covered by cartilage which articulates with the penticular process of the incus (anvil) bone.

STAPES NECK: A constriction between the crura bone and stapes head. Here the tendon of the stapedius muscle is inserted.

STAPES TENDON: Tendon which holds the stapedius muscle to the pyramid of the posterior wall of the tympanic cavity (middle ear).

STAPES-TWO CRUA: The anterior and posterior processes or legs from the stapes bone neck and are connected at the ends by the stapes base, a flat oval plate. The anterior is short and curved, less than the posterior process.

STELLATE CELL: A star-shaped cell with a number of filaments traveling in all directions.

STENOSIS: A constriction or narrowing of a canal or duct.

STENSEN'S DUCT: (PAROTIC DUCT) Niels Stensen, Danish physician. Originates at the parotic gland, crosses the masseter muscle, passes through the buccenator muscle, and opens on the internal surface of the cheek opposite the upper second molar tooth. The duct is for secretion of saliva in the mouth.

STEREOCILIUM: A non-moving protoplasnic filament on the free surface of a cell. pl. stereocilia.

STEREOTROPISM: In embryo development, movement of organs and structures in response to coming into contact with a hard or rigid surface.

STERNOCLEIDOMASTOID MUSCLE: (STERNOMASTOID MUSCLE) A muscle of the neck and of inhalation. ORIGIN- From the clavicle and sternum bone. INSERTION- Mastoid process of the temporal bone. ACTION- Depress and rotate head. NERVE- Second and third cervical nerves.

STERNOHYOID MUSCLE: A flat strap-like extrinsic infrahoid muscle of the larynx. ORIGIN- Sternum bone manubrium portion. DIRECTION- Vertical. INSERTION- Hyoid bone body. ACTION- Depress hyoid bone and larynx. NERVE- Hypoglossal (XII cranial).

STERNOTHYROID MUSCLE: A long extrinsic infrahoid muscle of the

larynx. ORIGIN- Sternum bone manubrium portion. DIRECTION-
Vertical upward. INSERTION- Hyoid bone. ACTION- Depress thyroid
cartilage. NERVE- Hypoglossal (XII cranial).

STERNUM ANGLE: Angle formed between the sternum body and the
manubrium portion.

STERNUM BONE: (BREAST BONE) A flat oblong bone in the midline
at the front of the thorax. In the front it forms the anterior wall
of the thorax, and joining above with the clavicle bones, and on the
lateral surface by seven pair of indentations, for articulation of the
costal cartilage of the seven pair of true ribs. The lowest portion,
the xiphoid (ensiform) process, has no ribs attached but some abdominal muscles are attached.

STIMULUS: An act or influence that produces a reaction in a irritable
tissue or receptor.

STIRRUP: (STAPES BONE) The third and inner most bone of the ossicles of the tympanic cavity (middle ear). It articulates with the
incus (anvil) bone, and the stapes footplate inserts into the fenestra vestibuli (oval window). It consists of the head, neck, footplate,
and two crus (legs).

STOMACH TEETH: The lower canine teeth of the deciduous (temporary)
set.

STOMODEUM: (ORAL GROOVE) In embryo development, the infolding
of the ectoderm which forms the primitive mouth.

STOPS: Process where sounds are made by compressing the breath and
and suddenly releasing it.

STRAIN: Deformation produced by stress.

STRAP MUSCLES: Muscles which make up a portion of the hyoid bone
sling. Consists of the geniohyoid, omohyoid, sternohyoid, and
sternothyroid.

STRATIFIED; Arranged in layers.

STRATIFORM: Having a form of layers.

STRATUM ZONALE: A layer of white nerve fibers coverning the dorsal
surface of the thalamus, a portion of the forebrain.

STRESS: The action of forces whereby deformation or strain results.

STRETCH RECEPTOR: A propioceptor, consisting of a spindle of both motor and sensory fibers, receptive to change in luscle length.

STRIA: A line or streak. 2. A bandlike structure to designate a group of nerve fibers in the brain. pl. striae.

STRIA VASCULARIS: A layer of fibrous vascular tissue. It covers the outer wall of the cochlea duct, which secrests endolymph fluid, through which the organ of Corti receives nutrition.

STRIATED: Characterized by parallel-placed transverse fibers.

STRIATED: (STRIDED, SKELETAL) (VOLUNTARY MUSCLE) Muscle which is under conscious control. Consists of fibers grouped into bundles, or fasciculi covered by a sheath of connective tissue. It is found in the pharynx, skeletal muscles, tongue, and the superior portion of the esophagus.

STROBOLARYNGOSCOPY: Examination of the larynx, utilizing a stroboscope for illumination. When the rate of the flashing light is equal to that of the vibrating vocal folds, they seemingly stand motionless, thus affording a critical view.

STYLOGLOSSUS MUSCLE: An extrinsic muscle of the tongue. ORIGIN- Anterior of the styloid process. DIRECTION- Downward, lateral. INSERTION- Margin of the tongue. ACTION- Raise and retract tongue. NERVE- Hypoglossal (XII cranial).

STYLOHYAL: The styloid process and hyoid bone.

STYLOHYOID LIGAMENT: Elastic fibrous tissue from the hyoid bone lesser horn to the temporal bone styloid process.

STYLOHYOID MUSCLE: A long thin extrinsic suprahyoid muscle of the larynx. ORIGIN- Temporal bone, styloid process. DIRECTION- Downward and forward. INSERTION- Hyoid bone body near the greater cornu. ACTION- Draws hyoid bone and tongue upward. NERVE- Facial (VII cranial).

STYLOHYOID NERVE BRANCH: A motor branch of the facial (VII cranial) nerve, directed to the stylohyoid muscle.

STYLOID: Long and pointed, like a pillar.

STYLOID PROCESS- TEMPORAL BONE: A thin projection pointed downward from the inferior of the temporal bone. It serves for attachment for the styloglossus, stylohyoideus, and stylopharyngeus muscles and the stylohyoid and styomandibular ligaments.

STYLOMANDIBULAR LIGAMENT: A line of fascia extending from the posterior border of the mandible bone ramus to the styloid process of the temporal bone.

STYLOMASTOID FORAMEN: An opening in the temporal bone, between the mastoid and styloid processes, for of the facial (VII cranial) nerve and stylomastoid artery.

STYLOPHARYNGUS MUSCLE: A muscle of the pharynx, a pharyngeal levator. ORIGIN- Temporal bone styloid process. DIRECTION- Downward. INSERTION- Thyroid cartilage. ACTION- Raise pharynx. NERVE- Glossopharyngeal (IX cranial).

SUBARACHNOID SPACE: The space between the arachnoid and pia mater layers of the meninges. This space contains cerebrospinal fluid.

SUBCLAVIUS MUSCLE: A muscle of the thorax and of inhalation. ORIGIN- Area of the first rib and the costal cartilage. DIRECTION- Lateral. INSERTION- Area where the clavicle bone articulates with the acromion portion of the scapula. ACTION- Raise rib and depress clavicle bone. NERVE- Cervical fibe and six.

SUBCOSTAL MUSCLE: ORIGIN- From the inner surface and lower portion of the ribs near the angle. DIRECTION- Downward and medial. INSERTION- Inner surface of rib two and three. ACTION-Draw ribs together and depress. NERVE- Intercostal.

SUBCOSTAL NERVE: The twelfth thoracic nerve.

SUBLINGUAL GLAND; The smallest of the salivary glands. Located between the mandible bone and the sides of the tongue.

SUBLUXATION: A incomplete or partial dislocation.

SUBMANDIBULAR GANGLION: (SUBMAXILLARY GANGLION) A ganglion located on the lateral surface of the hyoglossus muscle. Peripheral fibers supply the lingual, sublingual, and submandibular salivary glands.

SUBMANDIBULAR GLAND: (SUBMAXILLARY GLAND) One of three pair of salivary glands located partially above and below the posterior of the base of the mandible bone.

SUBMANDIBULARIS DUCT: (WHARTON'S DUCT) Thomas Wharton, English physician. A thin duct that drains the submandibular gland, opening at the side of the frenulum linguae.

SUBMAXILLARY GANGLION: (SUBMANDIBULAR GANGLION) A ganglion located on the lateral surface of the hyoglossus muscle. Peripheral fibers supply the lingual, sublingual, and submandibular salivary glands.

SUBMAXILLARY GLAND: (SUBMANDIBULAR GLAND) One of three pair of salivary glands located partially above and below the posterior of the base of the mandible bone.

SUBMUCOUS: A layer of areolar tissue under a mucous membrane.

SUBSTANTIA NIGRA: A layer of dark gray matter separating the basis pedunculi from the tegmentum. Extending from the pons to the subthalamus.

SUBTHALAMUS: (VENTRAL THALAMUS) A portion of the diencephalon below the thalamus. Responsible for the relay of optic and vestibular activities.

SUCTORIAL PAD: (BUCCAL FAT PAD) (PAD OF BICHAT) Marie F. Bichat, French Anatomist. A deposit of fat in the cheeks superficial to the buccinator muscle. This pad is prominent in infants and assists in the sucking action.

SULCUS: A furrow, groove, or slight depression on the brain. pl. sulci.

SULCUS LIMITANS: In embryo development, a groove on the inner surface of each lateral wall of the neural tube. Divids it into the alar and basal plate.

SULCUS TERMINALIS: A slight depression directed forward and lateral to each side of the tongue margin.

SULCUS TYMPANICUS: (TYMPANIC GROOVE) A shallow groove at the bottom of the inner bony portion of the external ear canal. The thick annulus (ring) of the tympanic membrane (eardrum) fits into the groove.

SUMMATION: The accumulation of a number of stimuli applied to a muscle, nerve or a reflex arc.

SUPARMARGINAL GYRUS: A convolution on the inferior parietal lobe which arches over the turned up end of the lateral sulcus.

SUPERCILLARY ARCH: A curved process on the frontal bone just above the orbit. Joined to one another at midline by the glabella, a smooth elevation.

SUPERFICIAL: (EXTERNAL) Toward the surface. 2. Farther from the midline.

SUPERFICIAL TEMPORAL BRANCHES: Sensory branches of the auriculotemporal nerve, a branch of the mandibular nerve, the third and largest division of the trigeminal (V cranial) nerve. Directed to the skin on the skull temporal portion.

SUPERIOR: Toward the head or upper end.

SUPERIOR CEREBELLAR PEDUNCLE: (BRACHIUM CONJUNCTIVUM) The lateral wall on each side of the cephalic portion of the fourth ventricle.

SUPERIOR COLLICULUS: One of two projections forming the upper portion of the corpora quadrigemina of the midbrain. Containing the integration centers for optic reflexes.

SUPERIOR CONSTRICTOR MUSCLE: (CONSTRICTOR PHARYNGIS SUPERIOR MUSCLE) A thin muscle of the pharynx. ORIGIN- Mandible bone and medial pterygoid plate. DIRECTION- Backward and medial. INSERTION- On the medial raphe of the posterior wall of the pharynx. ACTION- Constricts the pharynx. NERVE- Vagus (X cranial) pharyngeal plexus.

SUPERIOR CORNU: (SUPERIOR HORN OF THYROID CARTILAGE) The superior extension of the posterior border of the thyroid cartilage. It attaches to the major cornu of the hyoid bone.

SUPERIOR FRONTAL GYRUS: The convolution on the frontal lobe, located above the superior frontal sulcus.

SUPERIOR GANGLION: (JUGULAR GANGLIA) An enlargement of the vagus (X cranial) nerve in the jugular foramen. From here motor and sensory fibers communicate with the accessory (XI cranial), facial (VII cranial) and glossopharyngeal (IX cranial) nerves.

SUPERIOR HORN OF THYROID CARTILAGE: (SUPERIOR CORNU) The superior extension of the posterior border of the thyroid cartilage.

It attaches to the mjaor cornu of the hyoid bone.

SUPERIOR LABIAL NERVE BRANCHES: Sensory branches of the infraorbital nerve, a branch of the maxillary nerve, the second division of the trigeminal (V cranial) nerve. Directed to the labial
glands and skin of the upper lip.

SUPERIOR LARYNGEAL NERVE: A motor and sensory branch of the
vagus (X cranial) nerve. It further divides into the external branch,
directed to the motor fibers of the constrictor pharyngis inferior and
cricothyroid muscles, and the internal branch directed to sensory
fibers of the aryepiglottic fold, epiglottis, and mucous membrane of
the tongue.

SUPERIOR LIGAMENT OF THE INCUS BONE: A fold of mucous mem
brane connecting the end of the short crus (leg) of the incus (anvil)
bone to the fossa incudis.

SUPERIOR LIGAMENT OF THE MALLEUS BONE: (MALLI SUPERIOR
LIGAMENT) A thin strand desending from the roof of the tympanic
cavity (middle ear) to the malleus (hammer) bone head.

SUPERIOR LONGITUDINAL MUSCLE: A layer of oblique and longitudinal intrinsic tongue muscles. ORIGIN- Septum of the tongue and
submucosa. DIRECTION- Forward. INSERTION- Tongue margins.
ACTION- Shorten, turn up lateral tongue margins. NERVE- Hypo -
glossal (XII cranial).

SUPERIOR MEDULLARY VELUM: MEDULLARY VELUM) A layer of fibers
forming a portion of the fourth ventricle roof.

SUPERIOR NASAL CONCHA: The superior of two bony plates. They
project from the inner wall of the ethmoid labyrinth, forming the
upper boundry of the superior passage of the nose.

SUPERIOR NUCHAL LINE: A line on the occipital bone outer surface,
curving from the protuberance to the lateral angle.

SUPERIOR OCCIPITAL GYRUS: The convolutions of the occipital lobe.
Located superior to the lateral occipital sulcus on the convex surface.

SUPERIOR OLIVE: Small masses of gray matter in the pons directing
third order neurons upward to the lateral lemniscus.

SUPERIOR ORBITAL FISSURE: A long groove on the sphenoid bone
between the great and small wings for passage of the abductent (I

cranial), oculomotor (III cranial), trochlear (IV cranial) nerves. Also the first division of the trigeminal (V cranial) nerve, the ophthalmic.

SUPERIOR SURFACE- MAXILLA BONE: (MAXILLA BONE-OBRITAL SURFACE) The smooth and triangular-shaped area, forming most of the orbital (superior) cavity floor. The medial border articulates with the ethmoid, lacrimal, and palatine bones.

SUPERIOR TEMPORAL GYRUS: The convolution of the temporal lobe between the lateral fissure and superior temporal sulcus.

SUPPLEMENTAL AIR: (RESERVE AIR) (EXPIRATORY RESERVE) The air that can be forcibly exhaled, after a normal exhalation.

SUPPORTING CELLS: Consist of cells forming a framework supporting the organ of Corti. They include the border cells, cells of Henson, inner and outer pillars, or rods, and the inner and outer phalangeal cells.

SUPPRESSOR AREA: Area of the frontal lobe where electrical stimulation in suppressed, and then gradually spread through the cortex.

SUPRAHYOID MUSCLES: Extrinsic muscles of the larynx. Consists of the digastic, geniohyoid, mylohyoid, and stylohyoid.

SUPRAOBRITAL NERVE: A small sensory branch of the frontal nerve, the largest branch of the ophthamic nerve, the first division of the trigeminal (V cranial) nerve. It supplies the upper eyelid.

SUPRASTERNAL NOTCH: (JUGULAR NOTCH) The notch on the superior border of the sternum bone between the clavicular notches.

SUPRATONSILLAR FOSSA: The small space between the palatoglossal and palatopharyngeal arches above the tonsil.

SUPRATROCHLEAR NERVE: A small sensory branch of the frontal nerve, the largest branch of the ophthemic nerve and the first division of the trigeminal (V cranial) nerve. Directed to the lower and midale forehead.

SUPRAVERSION: The displacement of a tooth abnormally elongated from its socket.

SUTURE: A synarthrodial joint in which the bony surfaces are so closely joined by a thin fibrous layer of connective tissue that no movement can occur. pl. suturae.

SWALLOWING: The movement of a substance from the mouth through the pharynx and esophagus to the stomach. In the first stage the hyoid bone and tongue are moved upward by the digastic, geniohyoid, and mylohyoid muscles. In the second stage the larynx, hyoid bone, and tongue are elevated. In the final stage, as the substance passes through the pharynx, the posterior belly of the digastric and stylohyoid muscles elevate and retract the hyoid bone tongue base to complete the movement.

SYMPATHETIC DIVISION-AUTONOMIC NERVOUS SYSTEM: (THORA - COLUMBER DIVISION-AUTONOMIC NERVOUS SYSTEM) This portion of the autonomic nervous system is connected to the central nervous system by neurons in the gray lateral columns of the spinal cord, The sympathetic truck ganglion chain, and the great prevertebral plexuses. Distribution is to the arteries, cranial nerves, individual organs, spinal nerves, glandular tissue and smooth muscle.

SYMPHYSIS: The line of fusion of two bones at a joint of fibrocartilage.

SYNAPSE: (SYNAPSE JUNCTION) Point of contact between two adjacent neurons. Forms the place where a nervous impulse is transmitted from one neuron to the other.

SYNAPTIC GAP: (SYNAPTIC JUNCTION) A junction in a neural pathway between two neurons where a nervous impulse is transmitted in one direction.

SYNARTHRODIAL JOINT: (IMMOVABLE JOINT) Formed by fibrous tissue consisting of four types of joints; gomphosis, schindylesis, suture, and synchondrosis.

SYNCHONDROSIS: Type of synarthrosis joint. The cartilage is changed to bone before adult like, sometimes called a temporary joint.

SYNDESMOSIS: A joint restricted in movement because of connective tissue attachment.

SYNERGIST: A muscle that functions in cooperation with another.

SYNERGISTIC: The ability of a muscle to improve the effect of another muscle.

SYNOSTOSIS: The union of bones by osseous cartilage or fibrous tissue.

SYNOVIA FLUID: A clear, alkaline viscid fluid found in bursae, joints, and tendon sheaths.

SYSTEM: The combination of parts into functional unity.

T

TACTILE DISK: The expanded end of a sensory nerve fiber responsive to light touch.

TASTE BUDS: An oval shaped structure on the epiglottis, a portion of the pharynx and the surface of the tongue.

TECTAL RIDGE: In embryo development, a medial projection on the globular process.

TECTORIAL MEMBRANE: (CORTI'S MEMBRANE) The gelatinous membrane brane forming the roof over the organ of Corti and into which the cilia of the hair cells are projected.

TECTOSPINAL TRACT: A descending motor tract of the spinal cord from the inferior and superior colliculi. Forms the ventral longitudinal bundle supplying effectors for visual reflex.

TECTUM: (QUADRIGEMINA) The dorsal portion of the midbrain, consisting of the inferior and superior portions. 2. A rooflike structure.

TEETH: A set of bone-like, hard structures in the mandible and maxilla bones used for the mastcation process. They are especially involved in speech production of the consonant sounds, and are important in all sounds made. The eruption of the deciduous or temporary teeth, twenty in number, begins at approximately the fifth month and ends approximately the thirtieth month. The permanent teeth begin to erupt at approximately age six or seven, and continue to approximately the twenty fifth year.

TEGMEN: A structure that covers. Such as the roof of a structure.

TEGMEN ORIS: In embryo development, the roof of the mouth.

TEGMEN TYMPANI: (TEGMENTAL WALL) (ROOF) The roof formed by a thin layer of the temporal bone petrous portion over the tympanic cavity (middle ear). Seperates the middle ear from the meninges of the cranium.

TEGMENTUM: A coverning or roof. 2. The dorsal portion of the cerebral peduncle. Consists of fiber tracts, nuclei, and reticular formations.

TELA: A weblike tissue, 2. membrane like a web.

TELENCEPHALON: (ENDBRAIN) In embryo development, the anterior portion of the prosencephalon. The cerebral hemispheres and corpora striata develope from this. Together with the diecephalon it forms the prosencephalon.

TELOCEPTOR: A sensory nerve receptor that responds to distant stimuli which exist in the ears, eyes, and nose.

TELODENDRIA: (END BRUSH) The many highly-branched tiny filament terminations of an axon.

TELOPHASE: The fourth and last phase in mitosis (cell division) after anaphase when the daughter nuclei is formed, the cell cytoplasm divides into two daughter cells.

TELEPHONE THEORY: (FREQUENCY THEORY) Proposes that the basilar membrane of the cochlea vibrates as a complete unit like the telephone diaphragm. The analysis of pitch preception occuring not in the cochlea but in the auditory (VIII cranial) nerve by the frequency of the impulse directed in each nerve fiber to the auditory area of the brain, the transverse temporal gyrus, (Heschl's gyrus).

TEMPLE: (TEMPORAL FOSSA) The lateral portion of the cranium. Out- '. the frontal and zygomatic bones, and the temporal lines.

TEMPORAL: The lateral part of the head, above the zygomatic arch.

TEMPORAL BONE: A irregular bone on each side of the cranium forming the base and sides of the crainal cavity. Consists of five portions; mastoid, petrous, squamous, stympanic and styloid. The petrous portion contains the organs of hearing and equilibrium. Articulation is with the mandible, occipital, parietal, sphenoid, and zygomatic bones.

TEMPORAL FOSSA: (TEMPORAL) The lateral portion of the cranium. Outlined by the frontal and zygomatic bones, and the temporal lines.

TEMPORAL GYRI: The inferior, middle, and superior gyri on the temporal lobe lateral surface.

TEMPORAL LOBE: The lobe below the fissure of Sylvius, and in front of the occipital lobe. The inferior, middle, and superior horizontal convolutions serving auditory functions are located therein.

TEMPORAL MUSCLE: (TEMPORALIS MUSCLE) A muscle of mastication. ORIGIN- Temporal fascia and fossa. DIRECTION- Downward and converging. INSERTION- Mandible bone coronoid process. ACTION- Closes jaws, retracts mandible bone. NERVE- Trigeminal (V cranial) Mandibular division.

TEMPORAL NERVE BRANCHES; Motor branches of the facial (VII cranial) nerve. Directed to the anterior and superior auricular corrugator, frontalis, and orbicularis oris muscles.

TEMPORAL PROCESS- ZYGOMATIC BONE: A long, narrow tooth-like, process which articulates with the zygomatic process of the temporal bone.

TEMPORAL SURFACE-ZYGOMATIC BONE: A concave surface with a rough triangular area medially, which articulate with the maxilla bone. Laterally its surface is smooth and concave, containing near its center the zygomatiotemporal forament for passage of the zygomaticotemporal nerve.

TEMPORARY TEETH: (DECIDUOUS TEETH) (MILK TEETH) The first set of teeth appearing from approximately the fifth through the thirieth month which are shed and followed by the permanent teeth. The twenty teeth include two canine, four incisor and four molar in each jaw represented by the dental formula:

$$I \frac{2\text{-}2}{2\text{-}2} \qquad C \frac{1\text{-}1}{1\text{-}1} \qquad M \frac{2\text{-}2}{2\text{-}2}$$

TEMPORAMANDIBULAR JOINT: Consist of the articular tubercle, condyle of the mandible bone, and mandibular fossa of the temporal bone. It is a combination ginglymus and gliding joint. A depression may be felt between the condyle of the mandible bone and the fossa of the temporal bone in front of the tragus of the ear as the mandible bone moves forward when the jaws are opened widely.

TEMPOROMANDIBULAR LIGAMENT: (LATERAL LIGAMENT) Two short bundles from the lateral surface of the zygomatic arch, to the lateral surface posterior border of the beck of the condyloid process of the mandible bone.

TEMPOROPONTINE FIBERS: Fibers of the midbrain arising from the temporal lobe, and terminating in the pons.

TEMPOROZYGOMATICA SUTURE: (ZYGOMATICOTEMPORAL SUTURE: The line between the temporal bone zygomatic process and the zygomatic bone temporal process.

TENDON: A fibrous, connective tissue, conelastic, of tough cords of closely packed white fibers. Serves for the attachment of muscle to bone.

TENSOR: Any muscle that stretches, or makes tense.

TENSOR PALATI MUSCLE: (TENSOR VELI PALATINI MUSCLE) A thin muscle of the soft palate. ORIGIN- Auditory tube lateral wall and sphenoid bone scaphoid fossa. DIRECTION-Vertical downward and medial. INSERTION- Palatine bone horizontal portion and soft palate. ACTION- Opens auditory tube, tenses soft palate. NERVE- Trigeminal (V cranial) mandibular division.

TENSOR TYMPANI MUSCLE: A muscle of the tympanic cavity (middle ear). ORIGIN- Auditory tube opening cartilage edge. DIRECTION- Upward and lateral. INSERTION- Malleus bone manubrium portion. ACTION- Tenses the eardrum. NERVE- Trigeminal (V cranial) mandibular division.

TERMINAL BUTTON: (END FOOT) An enlargement of a fibril, at the point of synapse where it makes contact with another cell.

TESTER/OVARIES: Glands of the endocrine system. The testes produce testosterone, important in development of male secondary sexual characteristics. The ovaries produce estrogen, important for development of female secondary sexual characteristics, and progesterone which initiates the menstrual cycle.

TESTOSTERONE: Hormone produced by the testes for development of secondary sexual characteristics.

THALAMUS: The large, middle ovoid-shaped portion of gray substance forming a portion of the lateral wall of the third ventricle between the epithalamus and hypothalamus. It functions as the major relay center for sensory impulses to the cerebral cortex.

THERAPY: Treatment of pathological conditions caused by disease, injury, or malformation.

THIGH: (FEMUR) Part of the lower body between the hip and knee.

THIRD ORDER NEURONS: Nerve fibers directed from the trapezoid body and lateral lemniscus to the inferior colliculus in the auditory pathway.

THIRD VENTRICLE: A small narrow, irregular cavity below and between the cerebral hemispheres. It is filled with spinal fluid, and communicates with the lateral ventricles by the foramen of Monro, and the fourth ventricle by the aqueduct of Silvius.

THORACIC: Pertaining to the chest.

THORACIC AORTA: The portion of the descending aorta, dividing into the bronchial, esophageal, mediastinal, and phrenic branches.

THORACIC CAVITY: (RIB CAGE) The skeletal framework of the chest. Consists of the ribs (twelve pair of flat long curved bones), sternum bone, and thoracic vertebrae.

THORACIC NERVES: The twelve pair of nerves which serve the abdomen and thorax. The first eleven pair are the intercostals, and the twelfth pair the subcostal.

THORACOLUMBAR DIVISION-AUTONOMIC NERVOUS SYSTEM: (SYMPATHETIC DIVISION-AUTONOMIC NERVOUS SYSTEM: This portion of the autonomic nervous system is connected to the central nervous system by neurons in the gray lateral columns of the spinal cord, the sympathetic trunk ganglion chain, and the great prevertebral plexuses. Distribution is to the arteries, cranial nerves, individual organs, spinal nerves, glandular tissue and smooth muscle.

THORACIC VERTEBRA: Twelve bones of the spinal column, between the the cervical and lumbar vertebrae.

THROAT: (GUTTUR) The pharynx. 2. The anterior part of the neck.

THYMUS: A ductless gland of the endocrine system, located anterior and superior to the heart in the mediastinal cavity. Its exact function is in conflict, but is believed that a hormone is involved in the initiation of immunity antibody formation.

THYOHYOID MUSCLE: (HYOTHYROID MUSCLE) A extrinsic infrahyoid muscle of the larynx. ORIGIN- Thyroid cartilage, oblique line. DIRECTION- Vertical, upward. INSERTION- Hyoid bone greater cornu. ACTION- Depress hyoid bone or raise larynx. NERVE- Hypoglossal

(XII cranial).

THYROARYTENOID MUSCLE: Intrinsic muscle of the larynx which supports the ventricle wall and appendix. Being lateral and parallel to the fold and consisting of two portions, the thyromuscularis and thyrovocalis muscles.

THYROEPIGLOTTIC LIGAMENT: A fibrous band that attaches the stem of the leaf-shaped epiglottis to the thyroid cartilage below the super-ior notch.

THYROEPIGLOTTICUS MUSCLE: Nerve fibers of the thyroarytenoid muscle from the thyroid. Directed upward, inserting into the epiglottis margin.

THYROID: Shield-shaped. 2. A gland. 3. Cartilage of the larynx, shaped like a shield, that rests on the cricoid cartilage with an attachment for the vocal folds.

THYROID CARTILAGE: Two large plates of shield-shaped hyaline cart-ilage resting on the cricoid cartilage and forming the anterior and lateral walls of the larynx. The two plates are fused, forming a V-shaped notch, the adams apple, at an angle of approximately 120 degrees in the female, and 90 degrees in the male. An oblique line runs down and forward which serves for attachment of extrinsic laryngeal muscles.

THYROID FORAMEN: (OBTURATOR FORAMEN) The opening between the ischium and pubis bones.

THYROID GLAND: A ductless gland of the endocrine system. Located as two lobes, one on each side of the larynx, connected across the midline by the isthmus, a strip of tissue coverning the second and third trachea rings. The gland contains glandular tissue of closed follicles, containing colloid, a gelatinous substance which contains the thyroid hormone, thyroxin secreted by the epithelial cells. The thyroid gland is activated and regulated by the thyotropic hormone from the pituitary gland.

THYROID LAMINAE: Two plates of hyaline cartilage fused together to form the thyroid notch and angle, the adams apple.

THYROID NOTCH: A deep, V-shaped notch on the superior border of the thyroid cartilage of the larynx. Its formed by the incomplete fusion of two plates of hyaline cartilate just above the laryngeal prominence (adams apple).

THYROHYOID LIGAMENT: (LATERAL HYOTHYROID LIGAMENT) An extrinsic elastic cord-like ligament which suspends the larynx from the hyoid bone. The cord forms the posterior border of the hyothyroid membrane, and extends from the posterior tip of the greater horn of the hyoid bone to the tip of the superior of the thyroid cartilage. A small cartilaginous nodule may be found imbedded in the ligament.

THYROMUSCULARIS MUSCLE: (EXTERNAL THYROARYTENOID MUSCLE) A portion of the thyroarytenoid muscle, located parallel to the vocalis muscle inserting into the thyroid lamina.

THYROVOCALIS MUSCLE: (VOCALIS MUSCLE) A portion of the thyroarytenoid muscle forming a majority of the true vocal folds. ORIGIN- Thyroid cartilage, posterior surface of the angle. DIREC-TION- Posterior. INSERTION- Arytenoid cartilage, vocal process. ACTION- Shorten and tense the true vocal folds. NERVE-Recurrent laryngeal.

TIDAL AIR: Exchange of approximately 750 cubic centimeters of air during a normal breathing cycle.

TIDAL VOLUME: The volume of air inhaled and exhaled by an adult during a normal quiet cycle of breathing.

TIP; The end of the tongue, narrow and thin bearest the teeth, which is directed against the lower incisor teeth.

TISSUE: A collection or group of like cells and their intercellular substance acting together to perform a function. The elementary tissues are;connective, epithelial, muscle, nervous, and vascular.

TONGUE: (LINGUA) The organ of the mouth. Attached by mucous membrane to the mouth floor and by muscles to the epiglottis, hyoid bone, mandible bone, palate, pharynx walls, and styloid process. It is free to move anteriorly, dorsally, and laterally aiding in deglution, mastication and speech production. Its movement modifies the resonance characteristics of the oral cavity and in the production of voiced consonants. The tongue is divided anatomincally into the blade and root, and functionally into the back, blade, front, and tip. The surface contains papillae of three types; filiform, fungiform and vallate.

TONGUE MUSCLES-EXTRINSIC: Consists of the genioglossus, hyoglossus, and styloglossus muscles.

TONGUE MUSCLES-INTRINSIC: Consists of the inferior longitudnal, superior longitudnal, transverse, and vertical muscles.

TONSIL: A mass of lymphoid tissue forming a ring in the depression of the mucous membrane of the fauces and pharynx. The tonsils act against the invasion of the body by bacteria.

TONSILLAR FOSSA: Depression between the palatoglossal and palatopharyngeal arches where the palatine tonsil is located on each side of the oral pharynx.

TONSILLAR NERVE BRANCHES: Sensory branches of the glossopharyngeal (IX cranial) nerve. Directed to the fauces and soft palate.

TONSILLAR RING: (WALDEYER'S WING) Wilhem von Waldeyer, Anatomist. The ring of lymphoid tissue formed by the lingual, palatine (faucia) and pharyngeal tonsils around the pharynx.

TOOTH: One of a set of hard, bone-like structure in the jaws for the chewing of food, Each tooth consists of three major parts: the crown, above the gum; the neck, between the crown and root; and the root, embedded in a socket in the gums. A tooth is made up of a solid part and a pulp cavity. The solid part includes dentin or ivory, similar to bone but harder; enamel, which covers and protects the dentin and crown; and cementum, a bone coverning of the root. The pulp cavity inside the crown contains a canal with the root that opens at the apex for nerves and vessels. It contains dental pulp, a soft sensitive material containing cells, connective tissue, nerves and vessels.

TOOTH BUDS: In embryo development, the knoblike swelling in the dental lamina.

TOPICAL: Pertaining to a local, or special area.

TORQUE: The force produced in the rotation, or torsion of a body on an axis.

TORIVERSION; The displacement of a tooth rotated or turned on its long axis out of normal position.

TORSO: The body, minus the head and extremities.

TORTUOUS: Twist, turned.

TORUS: A projection or swelling.

TORUS TUBARIUS: (EUSTACHIAN CUSHION) A ridge of cartilage covered with ciliated mucous membrane behind the pharyngeal opening of the auditory (Eustachian) tube.

TRACHEA: (WINDPIPE) A cartilaginous horseshoe, or U shaped tube composed of sixteen to twenty rings of hyline cartilage, each separated by a fibroelastic membrane. Each ring opening lies toward the back where they are in direct contact with the esophagus. It extends from the sixth cervical to the fifth thoracic vertebrae. At this point it bifurcates (divides) into the left and right bronchi stems, one for each lung. It is lined with mucous membrane continuous with the bronchi and larynx. The inner surface is lined with ciliated (hair) which is in continuous motion, moving rapidly downward and upward slowly in a cleaning action for dust and mucous. The first ring is larger and is connected with the inferior border of the cricoid cartilage of the larynx by the cricotracheal ligament.

TRACT: A pathway or course, especially of nerves. 2. A group of structures with a specific purpose.

TRACTION: Drawing, or pulling.

TRACTUS SOLITARIUS: A decending tract for taste of the medulla oblongata of fibers of the facial (VII cranial), glossopharyngeal (IX cranial), and vagus (X cranial) nerves.

TRAGI LAMINA: Cartilage which gives shape to the tragus on the external ear.

TRAGICUS MUSCLE: A muscle of the external ear. ORIGIN and INSERTION- Outer portion of the tragus. NERVE- Facial (VII cranial) temporal branch.

TRAGUS: (BUCK) Gordon Buck, American Surgeon, A small, tongue-like cartilaginous projection in front of the external ear external canal.

TRANDUCER: A device that absorbs and emits energy, either in the same form or in another form.

TRANSILLUMINATION: Examination of the larynx by concentrating a spot of light on the anterior portion of the neck. The interior of the larynx is illuminated by the concerntrated light passing through the tissue.

TRANSVERSE: (HORIZONTAL) Anatomic plane, across, dividing into upper and lower parts.

TRANSVERSE FISSURE: The fissure between the cerebellum and the cerebrum of the brain.

TRANSVERSE MUSCLE: A intrinsic muscle of the tongue. ORIGIN- Medial septum of the tongue. DIRECTION- Lateral. INSERTION- Dorsum and margin of the tongue. ACTION- Narrows the tongue. NERVE- Hypoglossus. (XII cranial).

TRANSVERSE FIRAMEN: The opening in each of the seven cervical vertebrae for the passage of the vertebra artery.

TRANSVERSE PALATINE SUTURE: The juction between the maxillae bones palatine process and the palatine bones horizontal portions.

TRANSVERSE PROCESS: Extends dorsally and laterally from a vertebra arch.

TRANSVERSE SUTURE: (INFRAORBITALIS SUTURE) A fibrous joint directed from the infrorbital foramen to the infraorbital groove.

TRANSVERSE TEMPORAL GYRUS: (AREA 41-42) (HESCHL'S GYRUS) The auditory reception center below the Sylvius fissure of the temporal lobe.

TRANSVERSUS ABDOMINIS MUSCLE: A muscle of the abdomen and of exhalation. ORIGIN- Ribs six through twelve, inner surface. DIRECTION- Horizontal. INSERTION- Deep layer of abdominal aponeursis. ACTION- Compress abdomen and flex thorax. NERVE- Intercostals.

TRANSVERSUS AURICULAE MUSCLE: Muscle of the external ear. ORIGIN- Cranial surface of the ear. INSERTION- Circumference of the external ear. ACTION- Retracts the helix portion. NERVE- Facial (VII cranial) auricular branch.

TRANSVERSUS THORACIC MUSCLE: (TRIANGULARIS) A muscle of exhalation. of the thorax. ORIGIN- Sternum bone body and ensiform process and portions of ribs five through seven. DIRECTION- Upward and outward. INSERTION- Ribs two through six, lower borders. ACTION- Depress ribs, narrow chest. NERVE- Intercostal.

TRAPEZOID: A four sided figure with two parallel and two diverging sides.

TRAPEZOID BODY: A portion of the central auditory pathway. Consists of a group of fibers from the dorsal and ventral cochlear nuclei in the ventral portion of the pons. They cross at midline and turn at the superior olive of the other side to form a majority of the lateral lemniscus, and on to the inferior colliculus and medial geniculate body.

TRAVELING WAVE THEORY: Proposes that the stapes footplate causes a fluid wave to move along the entire length of the basilar membrane, with the amplitude riseing and falling. At the point of maximum amplitude the frequency of the sound is detected. Along the membrane the frequencies are highest near the fenestra vestibuli (oval window) and lower at the apex of the basilar membrane.

TRIANGULARIS MUSCLE: (DEPRESSOR ANGULI ORIS) A flat triang-ular muscle of the face. ORIGIN- Mandible bone ear the oblique line. line. DIRECTION- Vertical, upward. INSERTION- Mouth angle. ACTION- Pulls mouth angle down. NERVE- Facial (VII cranial).

TRICUSPID: Three cusps or heads.

TRIGEMINAL NERVE: (TRIGEMINUS NERVE) V cranial, A motor and sensory nerve with its origin in the brain from a large sensory and small motor root. The fivers of the motor root arise from two nuclei; superior, located in the cerebral aqueduct; and inferior, located in the upper part of the pons. The fibers of the sensory root arise from cells in the trigeminal ganglion in a cavity of the dura mater, near the apex of the temporal bone petrous portion. The fibers from the two roots combine into one, and then subdivide into three large divisions; the ophthalmic, maxillary, and mandibular. The ophthal-mic is a sensory nerve and is the smallest and divides into three branches; frontal, lacrimal and nasociliary. The maxillary, also a sensory nerve, divids into many branches directed to the dura mater, forehead, lips, teeth and gums. The mandibular is the largest div-ision and has both a sensory and motor function dividing into many branches directed to the lower part of the teeth, external ear, teeth and gums, muscles of mastication and a portion of the tongue.

TRIGEMINAL NUCLEUS: The group of nerve cells in the pons of the brain where the trigeminal (V cranial) nerve arises.

TRIGONUM: A small triangular shaped, cavity or structure.

TRIGONUM HABEBULAE: A triangular area of the epithalamus which receives olfactory fibers.

TRITICEAL CARTILAGE: A small, wheat-shaped cartilage nodule located in the lateral hyothyroid ligament.

TRITICEOUS: Shaped like a grain of wheat.

TRITURATION: Grinding. Toreduce to a power by grinding.

TROCHANTER: Either one of the two process below the femur bone neck.

TROCHLEAR: A structure shaped like a pully.

TROCHOID JOINT: (PIVOT JOINT) Type of diarthrodial joint which restricts movement to one axis.

TROCHLEAR NERVE: (TROCHLEARIS NERVE) IV cranial, a motor-sensory nerve with its origin just posterior to the inferior colliculus. It is directed to the anterior of the medullary velum, and across and cerebral peduncles, here they enter the superior orbital fissure, terminating in the superior oblique muscle of the eye moving the axis of vision up and down.

TROPHOBLAST: The outer layer of ectoderm tissue of the blastodermic vesicle. Attaches the ovum to the uterine wall and supplies the embryo with nutrition.

TRUE RIBS: (VERTEBROSTERNAL RIBS) The seven upper ribs on each side connected to the sternum bone by the costal cartilage.

TRUE VOCAL FOLDS: The two thick folds of mucous membrane which enclose the ventricular ligaments, narrow bands of fibrous tissue. They are located parallel to, and just under, the false vocal folds. The space between is the laryngeal ventricle. The folds originate from the posterior surface of the thyroid laminae, below the thyroid notch, below the angle and attach on the anterior-lateral surface of the arytenoid cartilage. The medial borders of the vocal folds are free so they project in a shelf-like manner into the larynx cavity. Earch fold is two bundles of muscle tissue bounded medially by the vocal ligament and covered by adherent mucous membrane. As air is forced out of the lungs it throws the two folds into vibrations, and the vibrations are transfered to the air above them and produce sound. The amount of force of the expired air determines, along with the range of the vibrations of the folds, the intensity or loudness of the voice. Voice pitch is determined by the number of vigrations made in a given unit of time dependent on the degree of fold elasticity, length, and thickness of the folds.

TRUE VOCAL LIGAMENTS: The free borders of the cricothyroid membrane.

TRUNK GANGLION: (CHAIN GANGLION) Nerve cell bodies in groups along the sympathetic trunk.

TUBER: A swelling protuberance.

TUBER CINEREVM: A small irregular shaped projection from the floor of the third ventricle between the mammillary bodies and optic chiasma. Bounded laterally by the cerebral peduncles and optic tract from a portion of the hypothalamus.

TUBERCLE: A solid, rounded elevation on a bone. 2. A solid elevation of the skin.

TUBERCULUM ACUSTICUM: (ACOUSTIC TUBERCLE) The dorsal nucleus of the cochlea nerve.

TUBERCULUM IMPAR: In embryo development, a tubercle at midline on the floor of the pharynx between the ends of the hyoid and mandibular arches.

TUBEROSITY: A round, elevated portion on a bone.

TUNING FORK: A metal fork with two prongs which, when struck, vibrate in a specific pitch of pure tone.

TUNNERL CELLS: (PILLAR CELLS) (RODS OF CORTI) Long cells which support the walls of the inner tunnel of Corti. The tunnel is formed by the articulation of the heads of the inner and outer pillar cells.

TURBINATE: Shaped like a top,

TYMPANIC ADITUS: The opening between the tympanic cavity (middle ear) and the tympanic antrum.

TYMPANIC ANTRUM: (MASTOID ANTRUM)A air filled, mucous membrane lined cavity anterior and superior to the mastoid porcess of the temporal bone. It communicates with the mastoid air cells and tympanic cavity (middle ear). The cavity is bounded by the tegmen above, moastoid process below, and squama portion of the temporal bone laterally and medially.

TYMPANIC CAVITY: (MIDDLE EAR) A small irregular cavity in the

216

temporal bone petrous portion. Contains the tympanic membrane (eardrum). The three bones of the ossicular chain, the incus (anvil), malleus (hammer), and stapes (stirrup), and the auditory (Eustachian) tube.

TYMPANIC GANGLION: Collection of nerve cells which separate from the glossopharyngeal (IX cranial) nerve .

TYMPANIC GROOVE (SULCUS TYMPANICUS) A shallow groove at the bottom of the inner bony portion of the external ear canal. The thick annulus (ring) of the tympanic membrane (eardrum) fits into the groove.

TYMPANIC MEMBRANE: (EARDRUM) A membrane which seperates the external auditory canal from the tympanic cavity (middle ear). The eardrum is disk-like, a three layer structure that extends obliquely downward and inward. The layers consist of the outer layer; a continuation of the skin lining the auditory canal; the inner most layer is mucous membrane lining the tympanic cavity; the central layer is fiberous, with fibers arranged both concentrical and radial that provides the resilient, thin connective tissue for strength. The top portion of the eardrum lacks the central layer and is lax, the pars flaccida. The rest of the eardrum has the central layer, being more stiff, the pars tensa.

TYMPANIC NERVE: (JACOBSON'S NERVE) Ludwic L. Jacobson, Danish Physician. A branch of the glossopharyngeal (IX cranial) nerve serving sensory and parasynpathetic functions, distribution to the auditory tube, mastoid air cells, and the tympanic cavity (middle ear).

TYMPANIC NOTCH: Located in the superior portion of the tympanic ring.

TYMPANIC PLATE: A thin plate of bone forming the floor of the tympanic cavity (middle ear), and separating it from the jugular fossa which holds the jugular vein.

TYMPANIC PORTION- TEMPORAL BONE: A curved bone located anterior to the mastoid porcess, and inferior to the squama portion. The anterior wall, floor, and a portion of the posterior wall of the external auditory canal, are formed by the concave posterior and superior surfaces. The boundry of the mandibular fossa being the anterior and inferior surfaces.

217

TYMPANIC RING: (ANNULUS TYMPANICUS) A fibrocartilaginous ring forming a portion of the temporal bone which develops into the pare tympanica of the bone by which the tympanic membrane (eardrum) is held in place.

TYMPANIC SULCUS: A groove in the external canal of the temporal bone which holds the tympanic membrane (eardrum).

TYMPANOMASTOIDEA FISSURE: (AURICULAR FISSURE) A groove in the temporal bone petrous portion between the mastoid and tympanic portions.

TYMPANUM: The middle ear, or tympanic cavity.

TYPE I GOLGI CELLS: Nerve cells which have long axons passing out of the gray matter.

TYPE II GOLGI CELLS: Nerve cells which have short axons and do not pass out of the gray matter.

U

UMBILOCUS: The navel, or central abdominal depression at the region of attachment of the umbilical cord.

UMBO: The projecting center of a round surface.

UMBO OF TYMPANIC MEMBRANE: The central depressed portion of the deeply concave surface of the tympanic membrane (eardrum).

UNCIFORM: Being hook-shaped.

UNIPOLAR: Having only one pole, or process.

UNIPOLAR NEURON: A neuron cell body having only one axon.

UNSTRIATED MUSCLE: See INVOLUNTARY MUSCLE.

UPPER JAW BONE: (MAXILLA BONE) See MAXILLA BONE.

URANISCUS: The palate, or roof of the mouth.

UTRICLE: The larger of the two sacs of the membranous labyrinth, in the back and upper portion of the vestibule of the inner ear. A sensory area, the macula acustica utriculi, is in its wall. It communicates by five openings with the semicircular ducts. 2. a small sac.

UTRICULOSACCULAR DUCT: A duct connecting the saccule and utricle of the membranous labyrinth of the inner ear.

UTRICULOSACCULARIS: (SACCURAL DUCT) A duct which joins the saccule and utricle of the membranous labyrinth.

UVUAR MUSCLE: A muscle of the soft palate. ORIGIN- Soft palate aponeurosis and posterior nasal spine of the palatine bones. INSERTION- Uvula mucous membrane. ACTION- Raise uvula. NERVE- Vagus (X cranial) pharyngeal plexus.

UVULA: A small, cone-shaped process hanging from the lower border of the soft palate at midline.

V

VAGINAL: Sheath, or sheathlike structure.

VAGUS NERVE:X cranial, a motor and sensory nerve with its origin as small roots which exit between the inferior peduncle and olive under the glossopharyngeal (IX cranial) nerve. It is directed throug through the jugular foramen, forming the jugular and modose ganglia containing sensory cells. Smaller branches from the gang- ia are directed to the external auditory canal, external ear, dura mater. The pharyngeal branch is motor and sensory, directed to the pharynx muscles (except the tensor veli palatini) and the soft palate. The superior portion is divided into the external motor por- tion that supplies the cricothyroid muscle, and inferior pharyngeal constrictor, and the internal sensory portion that supplies the muc- ous membrane portions of the tongue base and supraglottal portions of the larynx. Below the larynx is the origin of the recurrent nerve, directed upward to terminate at the larynx. It supplies the muscles of the larynx, with the exception of the cricothyroid muscle. The left portion exits the vagus nerve below the right and ascends between the esophagus and trachea and through the cricothyroid membrane to the larynx. The right portion originates above the left, directed behind the right carotid to the esophagus and larynx.

VALLATE: Having a rim, or wall around a depression.

VALLATE PAPILLA: The largest of the papillae, numbering eight to twelve in an inverted V shaped row. Located on the tongue dorsum in front of the foramen cecum and sulcus terminalis.

VALLECULAE: Depression between the epiglottis and root of the tongue, on each side of the median glossoepiglottic fold. pl. valleculae.

VALSALVA'S LIGAMENTS: (AURICULAR LIGAMENTS) Antonio M. Valsalva, Italian Physician. The anterior, posterior and superior ligaments which assist in the attachment of the external ear to the side of the head.

VAS: A canal that carries a fluid.

VAS SPIRALE: A vessel in the basilar bembrane.

VASCULAR TISSUE: The blood bessels, heart, lumph, and their parts.

VEIN: Vessel that conveys blood toward the heart.

VELAR: Pertaining to the velum, or a veil-like structure.

VELOPHARYNGEAL SPHINCTER MUSCLE: (SPHINCTER OF WHILLIS) A portion of the superior constrictor muscle. ORIGIN- Soft palate at midline. DIRECTION- Horizontal backward. INSERTION- Pharynx median raphe. ACTION- Constracts pharynx. NERVE- Vagus (X cranial), pharyngeal plexus.

VELUM: See SOFT PALATE;

VENTER: (BELLY) The fleshy portion of a muscle. 2. The stomach.

VENTRAL: Away from the back, toward the front of the body.

VENTRAL COCHLEAR NUCLEI: The forward termination of the cochlear nerve fibers in the brain stem.

VENTRAL CORTICOSPINAL TRACT: (DIRECT PYRAMIDAL TRACT) A descending motor tract near the ventral median fissure in the cranial portion of the spinal cord. Origin is in the precentral motor gyrus, and is directed to the mid thoracic level.

VENTRAL FUNICULUS-ASCENDING TRACTS: (SPINAL CORD VENTRAL FUNICULUS-ASCENDING TRACTS) Consists of the ventral proper fasciculus and ventral spinothalamic.

VENTRAL FUNICULUS-DESCENDING TRACTS: (SPINAL CORD VENTRAL FUNICULUS-DESCENDING TRACTS) Consists of the sulcomarginal fasciculus, tectospinal, ventral corticospinal, ventral reticulospinal, and vestibulospinal.

VENTRAL HORN: (ANTERIOR COLUMN)(ANTERIOR HORN) Gray matter of the spinal column, wider than the dorsal horn, containing cells associated with motor functioning.

VENTRAL MEDIAL FISSURE: (ANTERIOR MEDIAL FISSURE) The deepest of the two divisions which divide the spinal cord into left and right halves. It contains a double fold of pia mater, with the floor formed by the ventral white commissure.

VENTRAL PLATE: (FLOOR PLATE) In embryo development, the longitudinal zone forming the neural tube floor.

VENTRAL RETICULOSPINAL TRACT: A descending motor tract of the spinal cord from the reticular formation of the pons. Directed to the majority of the skeletal muscles.

VENTRAL ROOT: (MOTOR ROOT) Originates from within the gray matter of the ventral columns of the spinal cord. They are motor fibers which form two bundles near the intervertebral foramen and transmits motor impulses from the spinal cord to the periphery.

VENTRAL SPINOCEREBELLAR TRACT: An asending tract of the spinal cord, arising at the level of the third lumbar nerve. Directed through the medulla and pons, to terminate at the superior cerebellar peduncle and vermis.

VENTRAL SPINOTHALAMIC TRACT: An ascending tract of the spinal cord from the gray matter of the opposite porterior column. Directed to the thalamus, sending tactile sensation of pressure and touch.

VENTRAL THALAMUS: (SUBTHALAMUS) A portion of the diencephalon below the thalamus, responsible for the relay of optic and vestibular activities.

VENTRICULAR APPENDIX: (SACCULE OF THE LARYNX) A small sac extending from the laryngeal ventricle, between the thyroarytenoid muscle and ventricular fold.

VENTRICLE: A small cavity. 2. Cavities in the brain forming continuous communication for cerebrospinal fluid.

VENTRICLE OF MORGAGNI: (VENTRICLE OF THE LARYNX) Giovanni B. Morgagni, Italian Anatomist. A spindle-shaped fossa located between the ventricular (false vocal folds) above, true vocal folds below, and the thyroarytenoid muscle laterally.

VENTRICULAR FOLDS: (FALSE VOCAL FOLDS) Two folds of thick mucous membrane above the vocal folds (true vocal folds). Each fold encloses a thin band of fibrous tissue, the ventricular ligament. The folds move with the arytenoid cartilages and are farther apart than the true vocal folds. They usually do not function in normal voice production, but function in holding of the breath, providing moisture for the true vocal folds, and protecting the larynx when swallowing.

VENTRICULAR LIGAMENT: (VESTIBULAR LIGAMENT) A narrow band of fibrous tissue located within two thick folds of mucous membrane, the ventricular folds. It attaches to the angle of the thyroid cartilage in front, and to the anterior lateral surface of the arytenoid cartilage above the vocal ligament. The lower border forms a free margin, the superior boundry of the ventricle of the larynx.

VENTRICULARIS MUSCLE: Fibers of the thyroarytenoid muscle from the arytenoid cartilage, inserting into the false vocal folds.

VERMILLION BORDER: The border of the facial skin with the pinkish area of the lips.

VERMIS: A wormlike structure. 2. The medial portion of the cerebellum, between the hemispheres.

VERMIS NODULUS: The point on the cerebellum area ventral surface for attachment of the inferior medullary velum.

VERSION, A turning, 2. A change of direction of an organ.

VERTEBRAL ARCH: Thoracic portion of a vertebra enclosing a vertebral foramen.

VERTEBRA: Consists of a body, or corpus from which two pedicles (legs) project posteriorly. From this a lamina like structure projects backward, fused at the midline, and form a neutral arch which enclose the vertebrae foramen that contains the spinal column. Two spinous processes are directed toward the back and inferior from this arch are attachment of ligaments and muscles. On each side a transverse process projects out laterally, forming attachment for ligaments and muscles. In the thoracic vertebrae these are articulation points for ribs. There are two inferior and two superior articular processes for vertebrae to form movable diarthrodial joints. Each type of vertebra has special identification points; cervical vertebra have a transverse foramen that contain arteries; thoracic vertebra have articular facets on the transverse processes, and vertebral bodies; lumbar vertebra have large bodies which do not contain articular facets on the bodies, transverse processes, or the transverse foramen. The sacrum is ossified intervertebral disk and form the base of the vertebral column. The coccyx is composed of small fused vertebrae which articulate with the sacrum.

VERTEBRAL: Pertaining to the vertebrae.

VERTEBRAL ARCH: (NEURAL ARCH) The arch of a vertebra formed by the laminae and pedicles.

VERTEBRAL CANAL: The canal containing the spinal cord and its meninges. Formed by the foramina of the vertebral column.

VERTEBRAL COLUMN: (BACKBONE) (SPINE) The portion of the axial skeleton, from the coccyx to the cranium, consisting of the coccyx, sacrum and five lumbar, twelve thoracic and seven cervical vertebra enclosing and protecting the spinal cord.

VERTEBRAL FORAMEN: Hollow space enclosed by the vertebral arch.

VERTEBRAL NOTCH: On the inferior surface of the vertebral arch for communication of a spinal nerve.

VERTEBRAL RIBS: (FLOATING RIBS) Two lower ribs, numbers eleven and twelve, not attached to the sternum bone by costal cartilage.

VERTEBROCHONDRAL: Consisting of a costal cartilage and a vertebra.

VERTEBROCHONDRAL RIBS: The five lower ribs on each side, not directly attached to the sternum bone.

VERTEBROCOSTAL: Consisting of a rib and a vertebra.

VERTEBROSTERNAL: Consisting of the sternum bone and vertebrae.

VERTEBROSTERNAL RIBS: (TRUE RIBS) The seven upper ribs on each side connected to the sternum bone by costal cartilage.

VERTEX: The top of the head. 2. The top most part.

VERTICAL PLATE: (PERPENDICULAR PLATE-ETHMOID BONE) A flat, thin polygonal-shaped plate descending from the under surface of the ethmoid bone cribriform plate forming a portion of the nasal septum and deflected to one side slightly. The anterior border articulates with the crest of the nasal bones and spine of the frontal bone. The inferior border serves for the attachment of the septal cartilage of the nose.

VERTICALIS MUSCLE: A intrinsic muscle of the tongue. ORIGIN- Mucous membrane of the tongue dorsum. DIRECTION- Downward and lateral. INSERTION- Base and sides of tongue. ACTION- Pulls tongue flat. NERVE- Hypoglossal (XII cranial).

VESICLE: A small sac containing fluid.

VESTIBULAR AQUEDUCT: Located in the median wall of the vestibule of the bony labyrith. It transmits the ductus endolymphaticus, a duct extending the labyrinth through which the endolymph fluid passes to the inner layer of the dura mater in the cranial cavity where it terminates.

VESTIBULAR CANAL: (SCALA VESTIBULI: The upper portion of the cochlea containing perilymph fluid. It extends from the fenestra vestibuli (oval window) to the helicotrema (tip) of the cochlea.

VESTIBULAR GANGLION: (GANGLION OF SCARPA) Antonio Scarpa, Italian Anatomist. The sensory ganglion of bipolar cells of the vestibular division of the acoustic (VIII cranial) nerve. Its fibers arise from the cristae of the ampullae of the semicircular ducts, saccule, and utricule.

VESTIBULAR LABYRINTH: Part of the inner ear which contains the saccule, semicircular canals, and utricle.

VESTIBULAR LIGAMENT: (VENTRICULAR LIGAMENT) A narrow band of fibrous tissue located within two thick folds of mucous membrane, the ventricular folds. It attaches to the angle of the thyroid cartilage in front and to the anterior lateral surface of the arytenoid cartilage above the vocal ligament. The lower border forms a free margin, the superior boundry of the ventricle of the larynx.

VESTIBULAR NERVE: A portion of the auditory (VIII cranial) nerve. Its origin is from the ganglion in the lateral end of the internal auditory canal. It further branches to the ampullae of the semicircular canals, and the saccule and utricle in the vestibule of the inner ear.

VESTIBULE: The middle portion of the bony labyrinth, Ovoid (egg-shaped), it is continuous with the semicircular canals and cochlea. The tympanic wall contains the fenestra vestibuli (oval window). The medial wall contains a number of small perforations and the opening of the vestibular aqueduct. It contains a complex arrangment of chambers that contain sensory end organs that respond to head position changes, and equilibrium, the saccule and utricle.

VESTIBULE: An approach.

VESTIBULE: (VESTIBULE OF THE LARYNX; The portion of the larynx above the vocal folds.

VESTIBULOCOCHLEARIS NERVE: (AUDITORY NERVE) VIII cranial, a sensory nerve with two divisions. The cochlea division for auditory functioning has its origin in the organ of Corti of the inner ear directed through the internal auditory canal to the inferior peduncle between the medulla and pons. The vestibular division, for body equilibrium has its origin from the cells of the vestibular ganglion in the lateral end of the internal auditory canal, directed to and entering the medulla oblongata. The branches are directed to the semicircular ducts, saccule and utricle of the inner ear.

VESTIBULOSPINAL TRACT: A descending motor tract of the spinal cord. From the lateral vestibular nucleus to the sacral level and forms a portion of the balance and reflex mechanism.

VIBRATION CYCLE-TRUE VOCAL CORDS: One complete cycle consist of the opening, closing and closed phases.

VIBRATORY MOTION: Back and forth movement of a mass, directed toward a position of equilibrium or rest. Measured as to amplitude, displacement, frequency, perior, and phase. When it occures in equal time intervals it is called periodic.

VIBRATO: The effect placed on vocal tone which adds expression and warmth to the tone.

VILLUS: Small vascular process or protrusion. pl. villi.

VIRILISM: Masculinity.

VISCERAL ARCHES: (BRANCHIAL ARCHES) (PHARYNGEAL POUCHES) In embryo development, five pair of arches from which face and neck structures are formed. The mandibular, or first arch, forms the anterior portion of the tongue, lower lip, mandible bone and muscles of mastication. The hyoid or second arch, forms the hyoid bone lesser cornu, stapes, styloid process and stylohyoid ligament. The third arch forms the hyoid bone, greater cornu and the posterior portion of the tongue. The fourth arch forms the thyroid cartilage and from the fifth arch the arytenoid and cricoid cartilages are formed.

VISCERAL PLEURA: (PULMONARY PLEURA) The pleura which surrounds the lungs, and lines the fissures, and separates the lobes.

VISCOSITY: The property of a fluid which resists change in the shape, or arrangement of its elements during flow.

VISCUS: Generic term for the organs of any large body cavity. pl. viscera.

VITAL CAPACITY: The total amount of expiratory, inspiratory, and tidal volumes of air that can be exhaled after the deepest inhalation as possible.

VOCAL FOLDS: See TRUE VOCAL FOLDS.

VOCAL FOLDS-VIBRATION CYCLE: Consists of three phases; opening, closing, and closed.

VOCAL FOLD VIBRATION RATE: The rate is expressed either as fundamental frequency (hertz), or musical notes (pitch).

VOCAL GLOTTIS: (MEMBRANOUS GLOTTIS) The anterior three-fifths of the rima glottis. Bounded laterally by the muscular portion of the true vocal folds. It extends from the anterior commissure of the true vocal fold to the vocal process of the arytenoid cartilage.

VOCAL LIGAMENTS: The free border of the cricothryoid elastic membrane from the thyroid cartilage in front, to the vocal process of the arytenoid cartilage behind, in the vocal fold, forming the medial portion.

VOCAL MUSCLE: The inner portion of the thyroarytenoid muscle in the vocal lip in contact with the vocal ligament.

VOCAL PROCESS: The angle of the arytenoid cartilages, to which the vocal folds attach.

VOCAL TRACT: Consists of the buccal, nasal, oral, and pharyngeal

226

cavities. Acts as a generator and midifier of speech sounds.

VOCALIS MUSCLE: (THYROVOCALIS MUSCLE) A portion of the thyroarytenoid muscle forming a majority of the true vocal folds. ORIGIN-
Thyroid cartilage, posterior surface of the angle. DIRECTION- Posterior. INSERTION- Arytenoid cartilage, vocal process. ACTION- Shor
Shorten and tense the true vocal folds. NERVE- Recurrent laryngeal.

VOICEBOX: The larynx.

VOICED CONSONANTS: Consosant produced with vocal fold vibration.

VOICELESS or UNVOICED CONSONANTS: Consonant produced without the vocal fold vibration.

VOICE REGISTER: A series of succeeding sounds, on a scale from low
to high, of ewual quality made by the application of the same mechanical prinicipe The nature of the mechanical principle, which
differs basically from another series of succeeding sounds of equal
quality produced by another mechanical principle. 2. A series of
tones of human voice produced in the same way with the same
quality.

VOIT'S NERVE: A small branch of the auditory (VIII cranial) nerve
directed to the saccule.

VOLLEY THEORY: Proposes that when the nerve fibers along the
basilar membrane of the cochlea reach the area of maximum response a group of fibers act at a high frequency to fire in synchronous volleys by firing in small groups to match the upper limit need-
ed; as for a frequency of 2000 Hz there is synchronous firing of
four groups at 500Hz.

VOLUNTARY MUSCLE: (SKELETAL: STRIATED: STRIDED) Muscle which
is under conscious control. Consists of fibers grouped into bundles
or fasciculi covered by a sheath of connective tissue. It is found in
the larynx, skeletal muscles, tongue and the superior portion of the
esophagus.

VOMBER BONE: A thin, plowshare-shaped bone forming the lower
and posterior portion of the nasal septum, The anterior border
articulates with the cartilage portion of the nose, and the posterior
border is free. It articulates with the ethmoid bone perpendicular
plate, maxilla, palatine, and sphenoid bones.

VOWELS: (CARDINAL VOWELS) A set of sounds with preceptual quality the same, reguardless of the language. They are the descriptive physiological limits of tongue positions for the vowel sounds.

W

WALDEYER'S RING: (TONSILLAR RING) Wilhelm von Waldeyer, Anatomist. The ring of lymphoid tissue formed by the lingual, palatine (faucia) and pharyngeal tonsils around the pharynx.

WALLERIAN DEGENERATION: Augustus V. Waller, English Physician. The degeneration of the nerve fiber after separation from the cell body.

WAVE AMPLITUDE: The distance in height from the crest to the trough.

WAVE FREQUENCY: At a given point, the number of times a complete wave form passes per second.

WAVEFORM: The representation of a electromagnetic wave and the shape it displays.

WAVELENGTH: Thedistance between the crest (or troughs) of two sucessive compressions, representing one complete cycle vibration.

WHARTON'S DUCT: (SUBMANDIBULARIS DUCT) Thomas Wharton, English Physician. A thin duct that drains the submandibular gland, opening at the side of the frenulum linguae.

WHEATSTONE BRIDGE: An instrument designed to measure the electrical resistance of a component in an electrical circuit.

WHISPER: A nonvocal sound produced by the arrangement of the glottis during exhalation. The arytenoids are abducted and toe in so that there is a small triangular shaped chink in the area of the glottis. As the air stream is released, friction sounds are produced as turbulence occurs in the glottal chink.

WHITE COMMISSURE: The fibers which cross anterior and posterior to the spinal cord central canal from one side to the other.

WHITE LINE: (LINEA ALBA) A fibrous, dense white band of tissue at midline, extending from the ensiform process of the sternum bone to the pubic symphysis. The abdominal oblique and transverse muscles are attached nere.

WHITE NOISE: A sound containing a wide band of energy in all frequencies.

WHITE MATTER: Formed by white medullated nerve fibers.

WHITE RAMI FIBERS: Fibers which have their origin in the lateral gray portion of the spinal cord and thoracic nerves one through two or three. The fibers leave via the peripheral nerves and anterior root directed to the sympathic ganglia.

WINDPIPE: (TRACHEA) See TRACHEA.

WISDOM TOOTH: (MOLAR) The last tooth in the dental arch on each side of the jaw with a broad square crown and fused roots. They are the last to erupt, usually between the seventeen and twenty fifth year.

WRISBERG CARTILAGE: (CUNEIFORM CARTILAGE) Heinrich A. Wrisberg, German Anatomist. Two elongated, small yellow elastic cartilage one on each side in the aryepiglottic fold, appearing as small whitish elevations in front of the arytenoid cartilages.

X

X AXIS: The horizontal axis.

X COORDINATE: The abcissa, or horizontal axis.

XIPHOID: (ENSIFORM) Sword-shaped.

XIPHOID PROCESS: (ENSIFORM PROCESS) A sword-shaped cartilage process on the lower portion of the sternum supported by bone. No ribs are attached, only abdominal muscles.

Y

X AXIS: The ordinate, or vertical axis.

YOLK SAC: In embryo development, cells of the entoderm extending into the blastocyst cavity.

Z

ZONA ARCUATA: The inner portion of the basilar membrane which supports the organ of Corti.

ZONA PECTINATA: The outer portion of the basilar membrane, which is somewhat rigid and thick. A layer of vascular tissue is on the under surface. In this tissue a vessel, the vas spirale, lies below the tunnel of Corti, a part of the organ of Corti.

ZYGOMA: The zygomatic process of the temporal bone.

ZYGOMATIC ARCH: (CHEEK BONE) The formation of the zygomatic process of the temporal bone, and temporal process of the zygomatic bone.

ZYGOMATIC BONE: (CHEEK BONE) (MALAR BONE) Located at the lateral and upper portion of the face. Quadrangular in shape with processes of frontosphenoidal, maxillary, orbital and temporal, and the malar (outer) and temporal surfaces. It forms along with the zygomatic process of the maxilla and temporal bones, the zygomatic arch (cheek bone) and a portion of the orbital cavity lateral floor and wall. It articulates with the frontal, maxilla, spenoid and temporal bones.

ZYGOMATIC FOSSA: (INFRATEMPORAL FOSSA) An irregular shaped cavity medial to the zygomatic arch.

ZYGOMATIC MUSCLE: A muscle of facial expression. ORIGIN- The zygomatic bone in front of the temporal process. DIRECTION- Medial and oblique. INSERTION- Mouth angle and orbicularis oris muscle. ACTION- Pulls mouth angle back and upward. NERVE- Facial (VII cranial).

ZYGOMATIC NERVE: (ORBITAL NERVE) A sensory branch of the second division of the trigeminal (V cranial) nerve. It divides into the zygomaticofacial and zygomaticotemporal branches directed to the skin of the cheek and skin at the side of the forehead.

ZYGOMATIC NERVE BRANCHES: Motor branches of the facial (VII cranial) nerve, directed to the orbicularis oris muscle.

ZYGOMATIC PROCESS-FRONTAL BONE; A thick projection at the end of the supraorbital margin. Articulation is with the zygomatic bone.

ZYGOMATIC PROCESS-MAXILLA BONE: A rough, thrangular eminence articulating with the zygomatic bone. Located at the angle of separation of the anterior, infratemporal, and orbital surfaces.

ZYGOMATIC PROCESS-TEMPORAL BONE: A projection from the inferior of the squama portion of the temporal bone. The anterior portion articulates with the zygomatic bone temporal process.

ZYGOMATICOFACIAL NERVE BRANCH: A sensory branch of the zygomatic nerve, a branch of the maxillary nerve, the second division of the trigeminal (V cranial) nerve, directed to the skin of the cheek.

ZYGOMATICOMAXILLARY SUTURE: The line between the maxilla bone zygomatic process and the zygomatic bone.

ZYGOMATICOTEMPORAL NERVE BRANCH: A sensor branch of the zygomatic nerve, a branch of the maxillary nerve, the second division of the trigeminal (V cranial) nerve. Directed to the skin on the side of the forehead and side of the eye orbit.

ZYGOMATICOTEMPORAL SUTURE: (TEMPOROZYGOMATICA SUTURE) The line between the temporal bone zygomatic process and the zygomatic bone temporal process.

ZYGOTE: (ZYGOCYTE) A cell formed by two gametes.

I L L U S T R A T I O N S

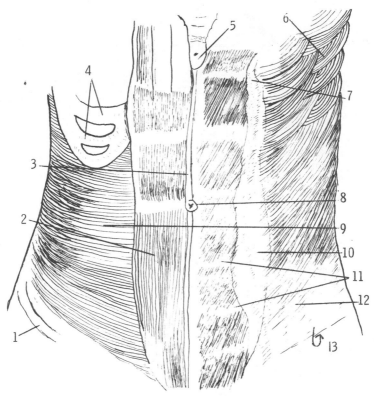

1 Iliac Crest
2 Rectus Abdominal M.
3 Linea Alba
4 Ribs
5 Ensiform Process
6 Serratus Anterior M.

7 Costal Border
8 Umbilicus
9 Transverse Abdominal M.
10 Linea Semilunaris
11 Tendonous Inscriptions
12 External Abdominal M.
13 Internal Abdominal M.

Abdominal Muscles

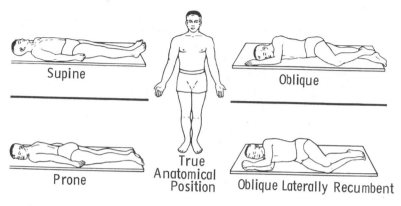

Supine

Oblique

Prone

True
Anatomical
Position

Oblique Laterally Recumbent

Movement

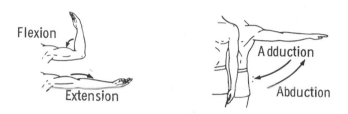

Flexion

Extension

Adduction

Abduction

ADDUCTION: Bending of head or trunk toward median plane of body.
ABDUCTION: Lateral beiding of the head or trunk away from the
median plane of the body.
FLEXION: The bending of a joint between the bones or a limb, decreas-
ing the angle.
EXTENSION: Straighting out of a flexed limb.

Body Movements

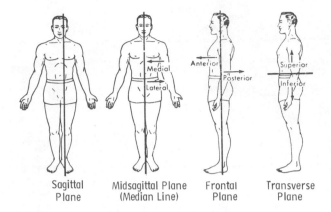

| Sagittal Plane | Midsagittal Plane (Median Line) | Frontal Plane | Transverse Plane |

PLANE	DIRECTION OF PLANE	DIVIDING INTO
Coronal	Side-to-Side (Lateral)	Front and Back Parts
Frontal	Side-to-Side (Lateral)	Front and Back Parts
Horizontal	Across	Upper and Lower Parts
Midsagittal	Front-to-Back	Equal Right and Left Parts
Sagittal	Front-to-Back	Right and Left Parts
Transverse	Across	Upper and Lower Parts

DIRECTION	LOCATION
Anterior	Toward the front or belly side
Caudal	Toward the lower or tail end
Cephalad	Toward the head or upper end
Cranial	Toward the head or upper end
Deep	Away from the surface
Distal	Away from the point of origin
Dorsal	Toward the back or rear end
External	Toward the outer surface
Inferior	Toward the lower or tail end
Internal	Toward the inner surface
Lateral	Away from the midline
Medial	Toward the midline or median plane
Mesial	Toward the midline or median plane
Posterior	Toward the back or rear
Proximal	Near the point of origin
Superior	Toward the head or upper end
Ventral	Toward the front or belly side

Body Planes and Directions

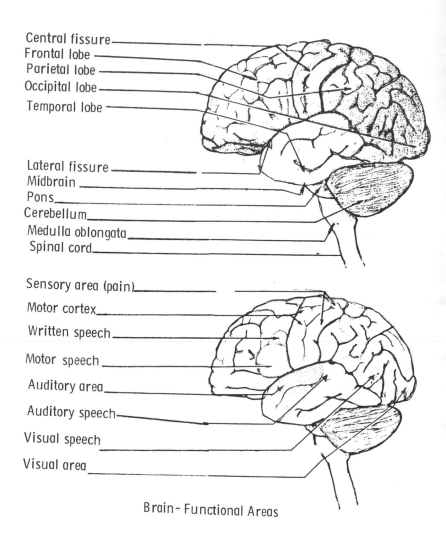

Central fissure

Frontal lobe

Parietal lobe

Occipital lobe

Temporal lobe

Lateral fissure

Midbrain

Pons

Cerebellum

Medulla oblongata

Spinal cord

Sensory area (pain)

Motor cortex

Written speech

Motor speech

Auditory area

Auditory speech

Visual speech

Visual area

Brain- Functional Areas

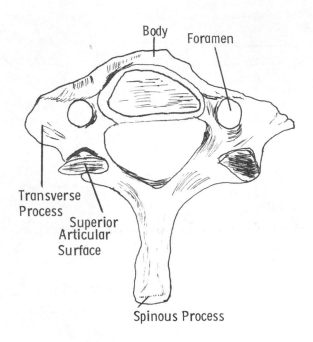

Body   Foramen

Transverse
Process
Superior
Articular
Surface

Spinous Process

Cervical Vertebra

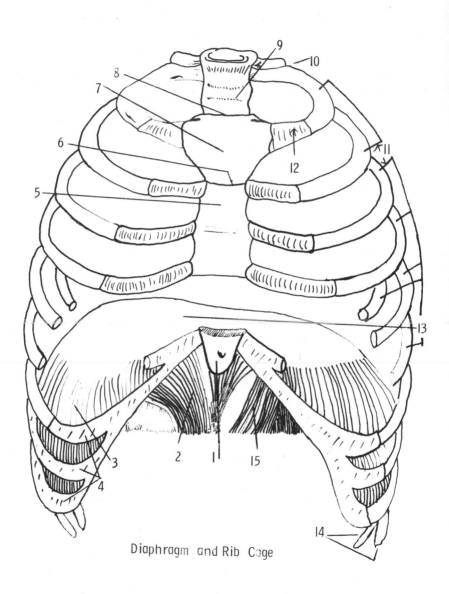

Diaphragm and Rib Cage

1 Ensiform Process- Sternum Bone
2 Right Crus
3 Diaphragm Muscle
4 Ribs, 8, 9, 10- Vertebrochondral
5 Sternum Bone- Body
6 Sternum Bone- Angle
7 Sternum Bone Manubrium
8 Jugular Notch
9 Vertebra
10 Rib Angle
11 Ribs 1 through 7- Vertebrosternal
12 Costal Cartilage
13 Central Tendon
14 Ribs, 11, 12- False Ribs
15 Left Crus

Diaphragm and Rib Cage Landmarks

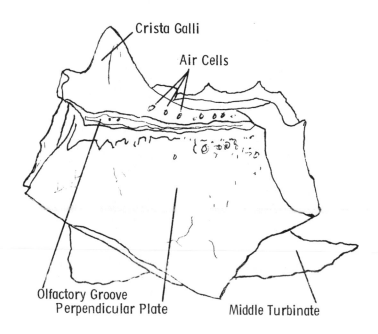

Ethmoid Bone- Lateral View (Labyrinth removed)

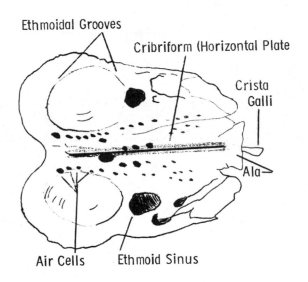

Ethmoidal Grooves

Cribriform (Horizontal Plate

Crista
Galli

Ala

Air Cells   Ethmoid Sinus

Ethmoid Bone- Superior View

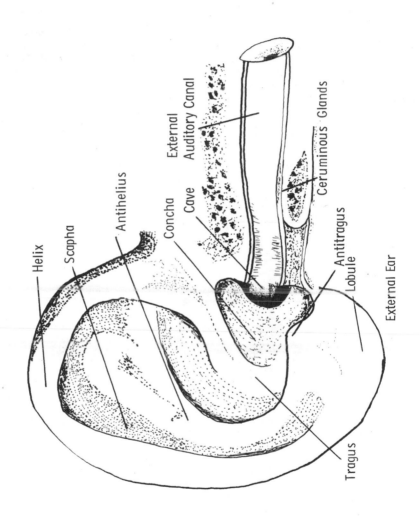

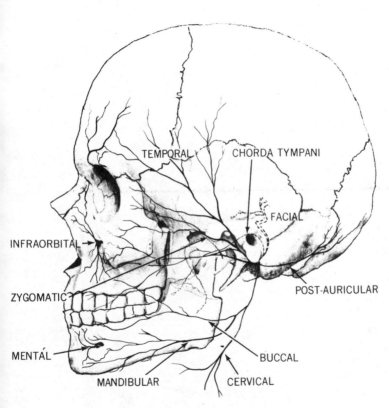

Facial (VII cranial) Nerve- Distribution

Forms and Shapes

Membrane	→	Membraniform	Almond →	Amygoaloiad
Moon (half)		Semilunar	Anvil	Incudiform
Needle		Acicular	Arrow	Sagittal
Nipple		Mastoid	Beak	Coracoid
Pea		Pisiform	Berry	Balliform
Pear		Piriform	Boat	Cymba
Pill		Bolus	Bow	Arciform
Pillar		Styloid	Bulb	Bulbiform
Pit		Fovea	Comb	Pectiniform
Point		Punctiform	Cord	Funiculus
Pointed		Fastigium	Crescent	Meniscus
Pulley		Trochlear	Cross	Cruciform
Ribbon		Habenula	Dart	Belemnoid
Ring		Annular	Ear	Auriform
Rod		Baculiform	Feather	Penniform
Rope		Restiform	Fungus	Fungiform
S		Sigmoid	Funnel	Choanoid
Saddle		Salla	Globe	Globoid
Saw-like		Serrated	Handle	Manubrium
Seed		Sesamoid	Hook	Unciform
Shell		Concha	Horn	Corniculum
Shield		Thyroid	Kidney	Reniform
Sieve		Gladiated	Kite	Rhomboid
Sickle		Falciform	Knuckle	Condyloid
Spindle		Fusiform	Ladle	Arytenoid
Spiral		Spiroid	Layers	Stratiform
Sponge		Spomgiform	Leaf	Folium
Spoon		Cochleariform	Leg	Crus
Sword		Ensiform	Lens	Lenticular
Tail		Cauda	Lip	Labium
Teeth		Dentiform	Loop	Fundiform

Thread	→	Filiform		Tree	→	Dendriform
Thorn		Spina		Web		Tela
Top		Turbinate		Wedge		Emboliform
Tongue		Lingua		Wing		Aliform

1- Rugae
2-Palatine Process Maxilla Bone
3-Transverse Palatine Suture
4-Horizontal Process, Palatine
5-Hamulus, Medial Pterygoid Plate
6-Posterior Nasal Spine
7-Lesser Palatine Foramina
8-Greater Palatine Foramen

9-Longitudinal Suture
10-Maxillary Premaxillary Suture
11-Canine Tooth
12-Foramina of Scarpa
13-Lateral Incisor Tooth
14-Incisive Foramen
15-Incisive Canal(fossa)
16-Incisive(Premaxilla Bone)

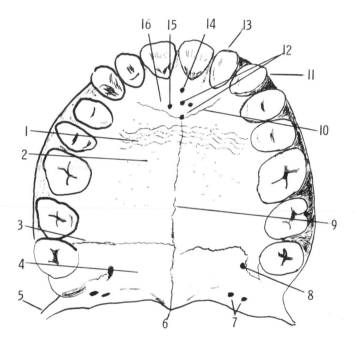

Hard (Bony) Palate

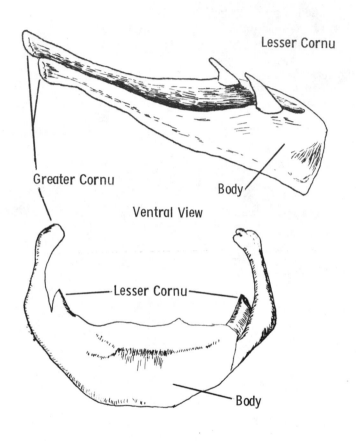

Lesser Cornu

Greater Cornu

Body

Ventral View

Lesser Cornu

Body

Hyoid Bone- Lateral View

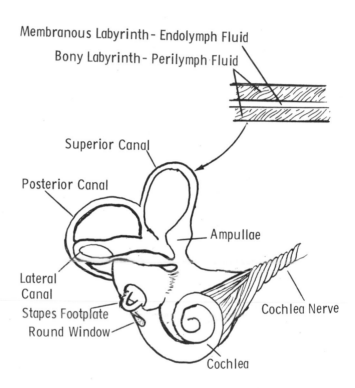

Membranous Labyrinth- Endolymph Fluid
Bony Labyrinth- Perilymph Fluid

Superior Canal

Posterior Canal

Ampullae

Lateral
Canal

Stapes Footplate
Round Window

Cochlea Nerve

Cochlea

Internal Ear

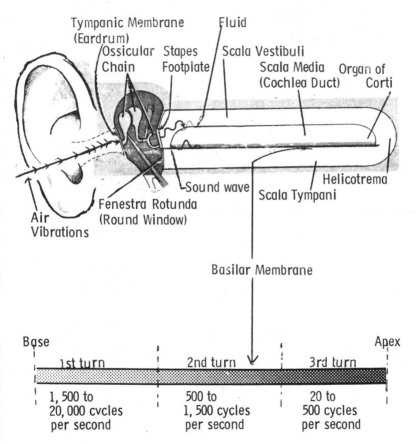

Tympanic Membrane
(Eardrum)
Ossicular Stapes
Chain Footplate
Fluid
Scala Vestibuli
Scala Media
(Cochlea Duct)
Organ of
Corti
Sound wave
Fenestra Rotunda
(Round Window)
Scala Tympani
Helicotrema
Air
Vibrations
Basilar Membrane

Base | 1st turn | 2nd turn | 3rd turn | Apex

| 1,500 to 20,000 cycles per second | 500 to 1,500 cycles per second | 20 to 500 cycles per second |

Internal Ear Hearing Mechanism

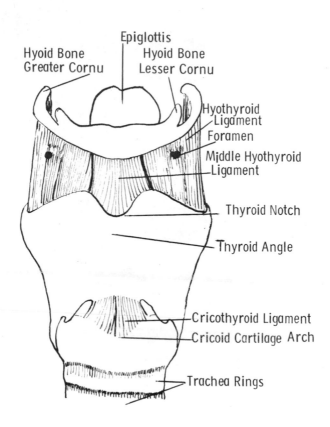

Larynx- Anterior View

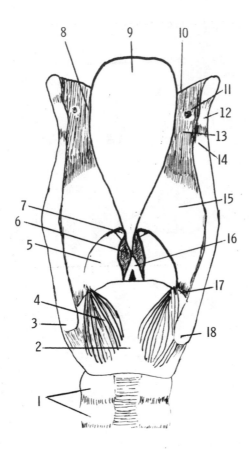

Larynx - Posterior View

1 Tracheal Rings
2 Cricoid Cartilage
3 Inferior Cornu- Thyroid Cartilage
4 Posterior Crico-Arytenoid Muscle
5 Arytenoid Cartilage
6 False Vocal Fold
7 Corniculate Cartilage
8 Aryepiglottic Fold
9 Epiglottis
10 Hyoid Bone
11 Foramen for Superior Laryngeal Vessels
12 Triticeous Cartilage
13 Thyroid Membrane
14 Thyroid Cartilage-Superior Cornu
15 Thyroid Cartilage
16 True Vocal Fold
17 Arytenoid Muscle Process
18 Thyroid Cartilage- Inferior Cornu

Larynx- Posterior View Landmarks

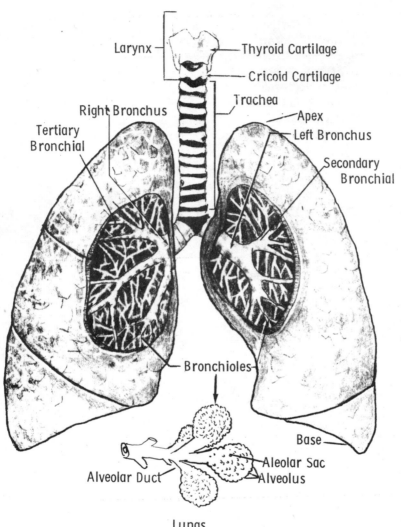

Larynx — Thyroid Cartilage

Cricoid Cartilage

Trachea

Right Bronchus

Apex

Left Bronchus

Tertiary Bronchial

Secondary Bronchial

Bronchioles

Base

Aleolar Sac

Alveolus

Alveolar Duct

Lungs

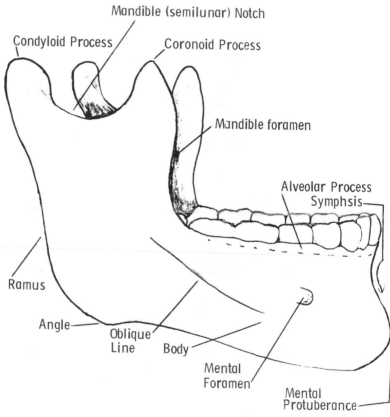

Mandible Bone- Lateral View

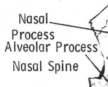

Nasal Process
Alveolar Process
Nasal Spine
Zygomatic Process
Maxillary Tuberosity

Lateral View

Frontal Process
Maxillary Sinus
Palatine Process

Medial View

Maxilla Bone

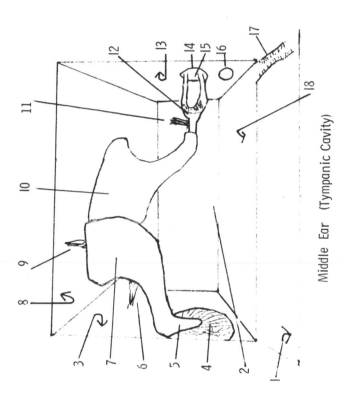

Middle Ear (Tympanic Cavity)

1 Carotid (Anterior Wall)
2 Mastoid Wall (Posterior Wall)
3 Membranous Wall (Lateral Wall)
4 Tympanic Membrane (eardrum)
5 Manubrium of Malleus Bone
6 Lateral Ligament-Malleus Bone
7 Malleus Bone
8 Tegmental Wall (Roof)
9 Superior Ligament- Malleus Bone
10 Incus Bone
11 Stapedius Muscle
12 Labyrinthic (Medial Wall)
13 Stapes Bone
14 Fenestra Vestibuli (Oval Window)
15 Stapes Bone Footplate
16 Fenestra Rotunda (round window)
17 Auditory (Eustachian) Tube
18 Jugular Wall (Floor)

Middle Ear (Tympanic Cavity- Landmarks

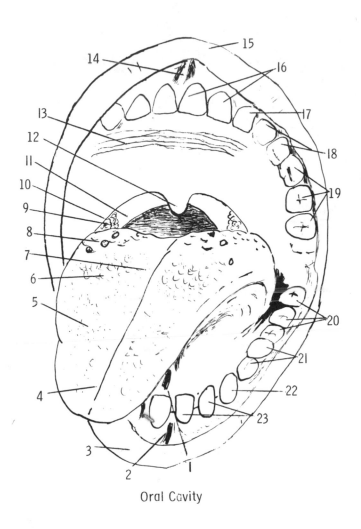

Oral Cavity

1 Lingual Frenum
2 Labial Frenum
3 Lower Lip
4 Median Sulcus
5 Filiform Papillae
6 Fungiform Papillae
7 Tongue Dorsum
8 Vallate Papillae
9 Palatine Tonsil
10 Anterior Fauce
11 Posterior Fauce
12 Uvual
13 Palate Ruga
14 Labial Frenum
15 Upper Lip
16 Incisors
17 Canine
18 Premolars
19 Molars
20 Molar
21 Premolars
22 Canine
23 Incisors

Oral Cavity Landmarks

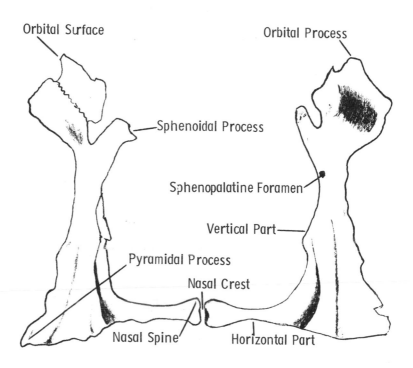

Orbital Surface

Orbital Process

Sphenoidal Process

Sphenopalatine Foramen

Vertical Part

Pyramidal Process

Nasal Crest

Nasal Spine

Horizontal Part

Palatine Bones- Posterior View

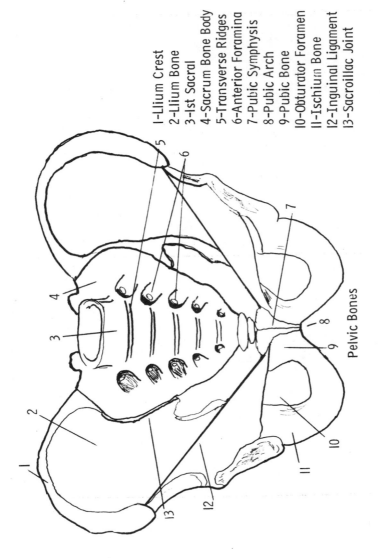

1-Llium Crest
2-Llium Bone
3-Ist Sacral
4-Sacrum Bone Body
5-Transverse Ridges
6-Anterior Foramina
7-Pubic Symphysis
8-Pubic Arch
9-Pubic Bone
10-Obturator Foramen
11-Ischium Bone
12-Inguinal Ligament
13-Sacroiliac Joint

Pelvic Bones

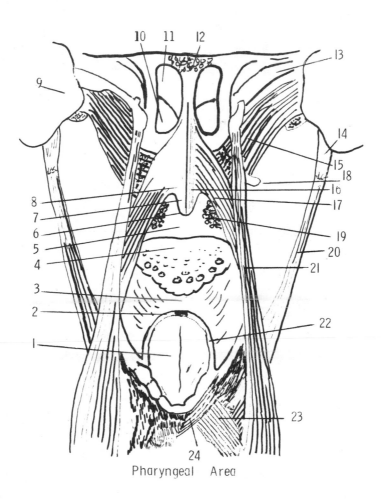

Pharyngeal Area

1- Larynx
2- Epiglottis
3- Tongue Base
4- Tongue
5- Oral Cavity
6- Uvula
7- Palate Velum
8- Soft Palate
9- Mastoid Portion-Temporal Bone
10-Inferior Concha
11-Middle Concha
12-Pharyngeal Tonsil
13-Auditory Tube Cartilage
14- Styloid Process-Temporal Bone
15-Tensor Veli Palatine Muscle
16-Uvular Muscle
17- Palatopharyngeal Muscle
18-Pterygoid Hamulus
19-Palatine Tonsil
20-Stylopharyngeal Muscle
21-Salpingopharyngeal Muscle
22-Aryepiglottic Fold
23-Arytenoid Muscle
24-Aryepiglottic Muscle

Pharyngeal Area-Major Landmarks

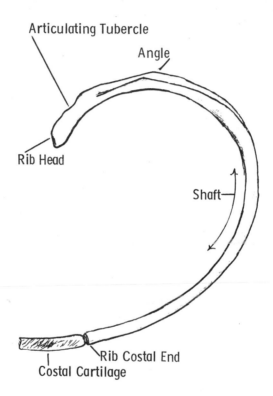

Rib

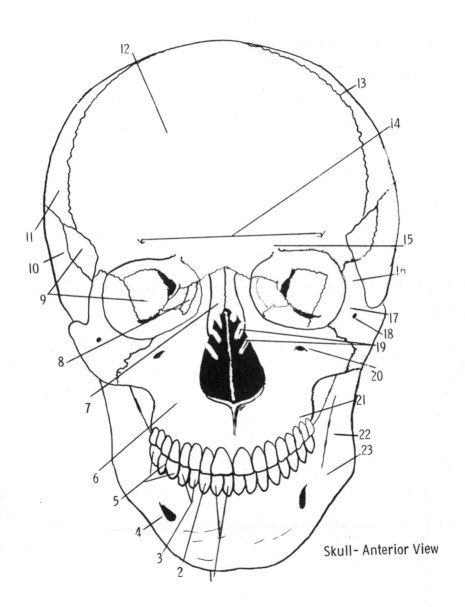

Skull- Anterior View

1 Incisor Teeth
2 Cavine Tooth
3 Premolar Teeth
4 Mental Foramen
5 Molar Teeth
6 Maxilla Bone
7 Nasal Bone
8 Lacrimal Bone
9 Sphenoid Bone
10 Temporal Bone
11 Parietal Bone
12 Brontal Bone
13 Coronal Suture
14 Oribital Paltes
15 Supraorbital Foramen
16 Zygomatic Bone- Frontal Process
17 Zygomatic Bone
18 Zygomaticofacial Foramen
19 Inferior Nasal Concha
20 Infraorbital Foramen
21 Maxilla Bone- Alveolar Process
22 Mandible Bone- Oblique Line
23 Mandible Bone

Skull Landmarks- Anterior View

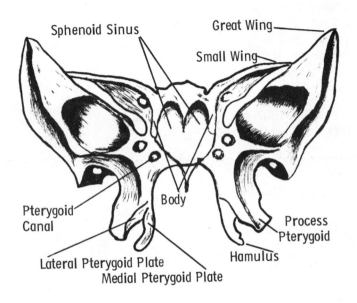

Sphenoid Sinus

Great Wing

Small Wing

Body

Pterygoid Canal

Process Pterygoid

Hamulus

Lateral Pterygoid Plate

Medial Pterygoid Plate

Sphenoid Bone-Anterior View

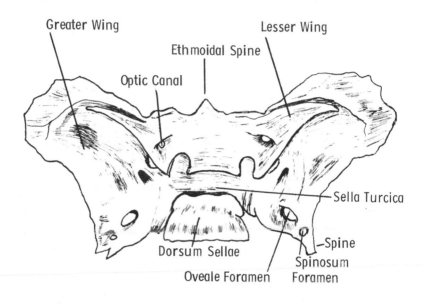

Sphenoid Bone- Superior View

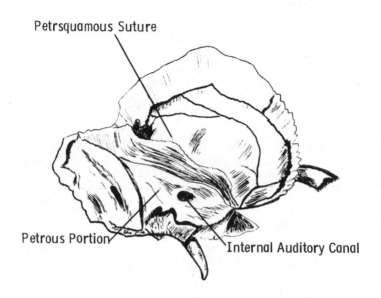

Petrsquamous Suture

Petrous Portion

Internal Auditory Canal

Temporal Bone- Inner Surface Superior View

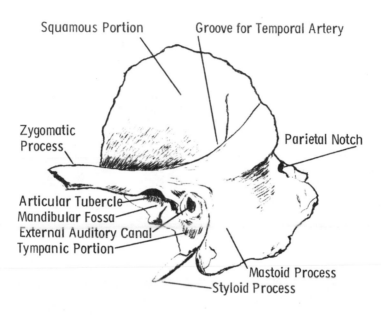

Squamous Portion   Groove for Temporal Artery

Zygomatic
Process

Parietal Notch

Articular Tubercle
Mandibular Fossa
External Auditory Canal
Tympanic Portion

Mastoid Process
Styloid Process

Temporal Bone- Outer Surface

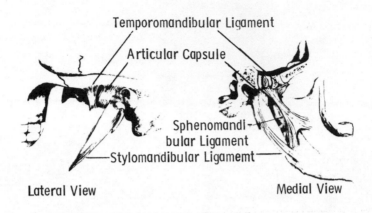

Temporomandibular Ligament

Articular Capsule

Sphenomandibular Ligament

Stylomandibular Ligamemt

Lateral View

Medial View

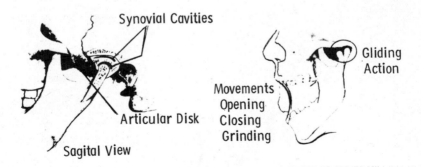

Synovial Cavities

Gliding Action

Movements
Opening
Closing
Grinding

Articular Disk

Sagital View

Temporomandibular Joint

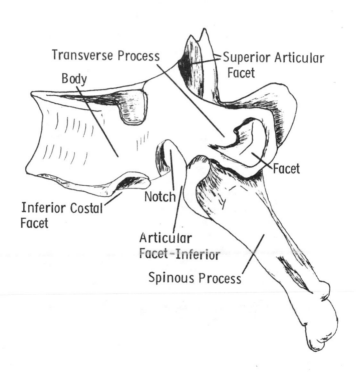

Transverse Process

Body

Superior Articular Facet

Facet

Inferior Costal Facet

Notch

Articular Facet-Inferior

Spinous Process

Thoracic Vertebra-Lateral View

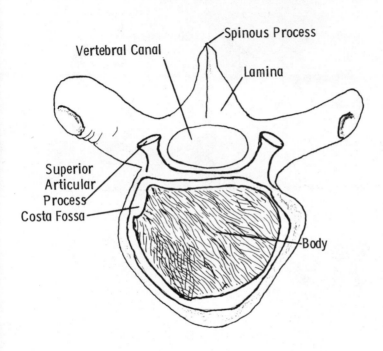

Thoracic Vertebra- Superior View

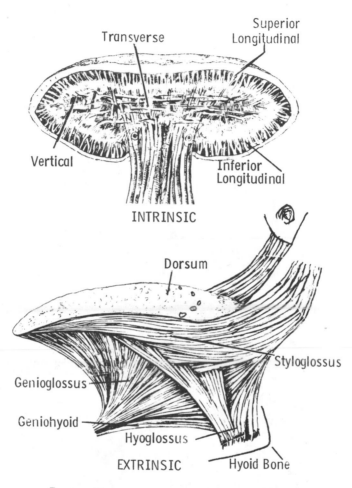

Tongue Muscles Intrinsic and Extrinsic

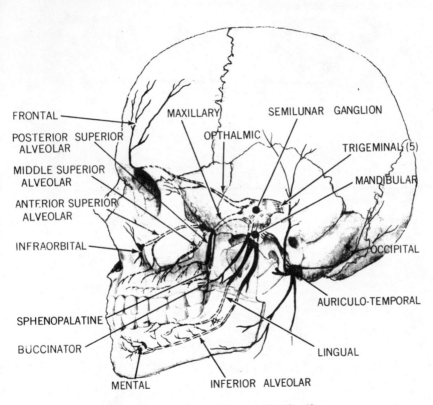

FRONTAL

MAXILLARY

OPTHALMIC

SEMILUNAR GANGLION

TRIGEMINAL (5)

POSTERIOR SUPERIOR
ALVEOLAR

MIDDLE SUPERIOR
ALVEOLAR

MANDIBULAR

ANTERIOR SUPERIOR
ALVEOLAR

INFRAORBITAL

OCCIPITAL

SPHENOPALATINE

AURICULO-TEMPORAL

BUCCINATOR

LINGUAL

MENTAL

INFERIOR ALVEOLAR

Trigeminal (V Cranial) Nerve- Distribution

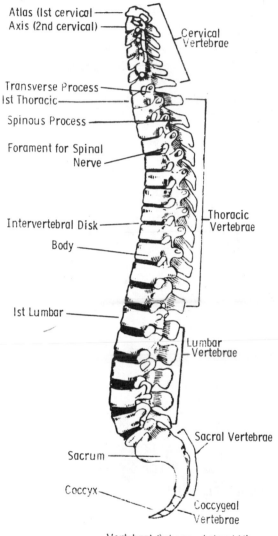

Atlas (1st cervical
Axis (2nd cervical)

Cervical
Vertebrae

Transverse Process
1st Thoracic

Spinous Process

Forament for Spinal
Nerve

Intervertebral Disk

Body

Thoracic
Vertebrae

1st Lumbar

Lumbar
Vertebrae

Sacral Vertebrae

Sacrum

Coccyx

Coccygeal
Vertebrae

Vertebral Column - Lateral View

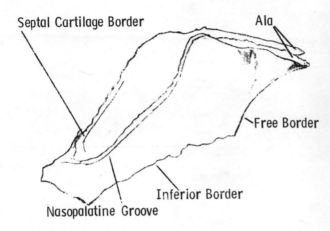

Septal Cartilage Border

Ala

Free Border

Inferior Border

Nasopalatine Groove

Vomer   Bone- Lateral View